"Democracy is more than a set of institutional rules; it is a collective psychological enterprise. This book bridges the gap between the clinical consulting room and the democratic town square to offer a profound diagnostic of our current age of polarization. At its core is the concept of mentalization—the essential human capacity to perceive others as complex, thinking beings.

Through a rigorous synthesis of attachment theory, developmental neuroscience, and an analysis of critical theory, the text demonstrates how the erosion of 'epistemic trust' has collapsed our shared reality, leaving us trapped in a landscape of tribal signaling. This is more than a theoretical critique; it is an urgent pedagogical roadmap. By advocating for a 'mentalizing stance' within our K-12 schools and wider communities, the book provides a verifiable path toward civic repair and psychological resilience. It is essential reading for educators, clinicians, and citizens seeking to understand the deep-seated psychological roots of our political fracturing—and how we might begin the work of building a more reflective and secure democratic future."

Harry Gill, *M.D., Ph.D.*

A Psychoanalytic Framework for Civic Renewal

A Psychoanalytic Framework for Civic Renewal: Reimagining Democracy from the Ground Up offers a compelling and original thesis: that the global crisis of democracy is not a purely political or economic problem but a deeply rooted psychological and relational one.

The book synthesizes key psychoanalytic and psychological concepts to argue that the health of a democracy is directly tied to the citizenry's capacity for mentalization—the foundational ability to understand ourselves and others in terms of our inner thoughts, feelings, and intentions. It methodically builds its argument, beginning with the developmental origins of mentalization in infancy and linking it to attachment theory and the cognitive function of theory of mind. It then expands this framework to the societal level, demonstrating how a collective failure to mentalize leads to the collapse of epistemic trust and a dangerous regression to primitive psychological defenses like splitting and "us vs. them" thinking. The work presents a powerful, integrated solution: a new educational model that cultivates not only mentalization and its core social–emotional skills but also the complementary intellectual capacity for critical thinking.

This book serves as a vital resource for educators, policy makers, and mental health professionals, offering an interdisciplinary framework that bridges the divide between abstract political theory and practical, psychological solutions.

Karyne E. Messina is a psychologist and psychoanalyst. She is on the medical staff of Suburban Hospital, which is part of Johns Hopkins Medicine. She is Chair of the American Psychoanalytic Association's Scholarship and Writing committee, which is part of the Department of Psychoanalytic Education. She is also a member of the President's Commission on Artificial Intelligence.

Dr. Messina has also written eight books and has three additional publications to be released in 2026 and 2027, focusing on applying psychoanalytic ideas to complex real-world issues we all face. She is currently writing a book, to be released this year, about the connection between mechanisms of defense—projection and projective identification—and AI bias, titled *Using Psychoanalysis to Understand and Address AI Bias: Refractions in the Digital Mirror.*

Psychoanalysis, Technology, and the Future Series
Series editor: Karyne E. Messina

Using Psychoanalysis to Understand and Address AI Bias
Refractions in the Digital Mirror
Karyne E. Messina

Madness and the Political Divide
Allen R. Dyer

A Psychoanalytic Framework for Civic Renewal
Reimagining Democracy from the Ground Up
Karyne E. Messina

A Psychoanalytic Framework for Civic Renewal

Reimagining Democracy from the Ground Up

Karyne E. Messina

Routledge
Taylor & Francis Group
LONDON AND NEW YORK

Designed cover image: Getty Image © Kubkoo

First published 2026
by Routledge
4 Park Square, Milton Park, Abingdon, Oxon OX14 4RN

and by Routledge
605 Third Avenue, New York, NY 10158

Routledge is an imprint of the Taylor & Francis Group, an informa business

British Library Cataloguing-in-Publication Data
A catalogue record for this book is available from the British Library

ISBN: 978-1-041-29772-7 (hbk)
ISBN: 978-1-041-29787-1 (pbk)
ISBN: 978-1-003-77129-6 (ebk)

DOI: 10.4324/9781003771296

Typeset in Times New Roman
by Apex CoVantage, LLC

To Dr. Wendy Jacobson

Training and Supervising Analyst, Professor of Psychiatry, mentor—and cherished friend.

Wendy, you exemplify the ideas at the heart of this book. While these pages argue for a democracy renewed through mentalization, epistemic trust, and civic empathy, you have long embodied these principles in practice—through your leadership, scholarship, and sustained commitment to the psychological foundations of social life.

I am deeply grateful for our journey together, which began at the American Psychoanalytic Association and grew into a collaboration marked by trust, intellectual generosity, and shared purpose. Your confidence in me, and your invitation to serve as Chair of the Scholarship and Writing Section for the Department of Psychoanalytic Education, provided both the opportunity and encouragement to refine the thinking that informs this work.

Alongside this professional partnership has been a genuine friendship—one grounded in mutual respect, curiosity, and care. Your presence has consistently expanded what felt possible, both intellectually and personally. It is an honor to dedicate this tenth book to you, in recognition of your mentorship, your ethical clarity, and the friendship that has so meaningfully shaped my work.

Contents

Preface

The profound challenges facing democracy today, from political polarization and the erosion of trust in institutions to the rise of authoritarianism, are often analyzed through political, economic, or sociological lenses. While these perspectives offer vital insights, they may not fully capture the deeply human dimensions of the crisis. This book ventures to explore a different yet complementary framework, positing that the current decay of our civic life is, at its heart, a psychological and relational phenomenon. It is a crisis of mind, not just of policy.

The Landscape of Civic Renewal: Why Education Is the Foundational Piece

To fully appreciate the urgency of the framework proposed in this book, it is necessary to situate it within the broader landscape of contemporary civic renewal. We are currently witnessing a proliferation of vital efforts designed to bandage our fractured democracy. Political scientists are proposing structural reforms to voting systems and legislative processes to reduce polarization. Community organizers and nonprofit leaders are tirelessly facilitating "bridge-building" dialogues, attempting to bring red and blue voters into rooms where they can see one another's humanity. Media literacy campaigns are launching public awareness initiatives to help adults spot disinformation and resist algorithmic manipulation.

These efforts are noble, necessary, and often heroic. However, they share a common, critical limitation: they are largely remedial. They attempt to "fix" in adults a set of psychological capacities that should have been built in childhood. Trying to teach a polarized, anxious, and epistemically mistrustful adult to engage in nuanced debate is akin to teaching a person to run a marathon after their muscles have already atrophied. It is possible, but it is arduous, resource-intensive, and often yields limited results because the underlying psychological infrastructure—the capacity to mentalize and trust—is already compromised.

This book posits that the most effective leverage point for democratic renewal is not in the repair of the adult polity but in the formation of the future citizen. The K-12 curriculum proposed herein is not intended to replace the work of policy makers or community organizers but to make their work possible. By embedding the skills of mentalization, epistemic trust, and critical thinking into the developmental DNA of the next generation, we aim to produce citizens for whom "bridge-building" is not a painful, artificial exercise but a natural psychological reflex. In this sense, the educational framework outlined in the following chapters serves as the foundational, long-term solution that undergirds and amplifies all other efforts to save our democracy.

This work draws upon contemporary psychoanalytic and psychological thinking to argue that the health of a democracy is predicated on the emotional and relational capacities of its citizenry. Specifically, it diagnoses a widespread and collective failure in the capacity to mentalize—the ability to understand ourselves and others in terms of our inner thoughts, feelings, and intentions. This deficit has led to a collapse of epistemic trust, leaving us isolated in ideological fortresses where shared truth and a sense of community become impossible. The paper further explores the psychological mechanisms at play, such as collective splitting and regression to primitive modes of functioning, which prevent citizens from tolerating the ambiguity and complexity essential for democratic deliberation.

By examining how core psychological concepts like mentalization, attachment, and epistemic trust are formed and how their absence can be collectively exploited, this paper aims to provide a nuanced understanding of our current political moment. It does not seek to replace existing analyses but to enrich them, offering a path forward that focuses on rebuilding the psychological foundations necessary for informed, empathetic, and truly engaged citizenship.

Introduction

Democracy today is grappling with profound challenges, from political polarization to the erosion of trust in its core institutions. While these issues are often understood through political or economic frameworks, this work posits a complementary and crucial lens: the psychological health of the citizenry. The crisis, as this book will argue, is one of the mind, a collective unraveling of the psychological and relational capacities essential for civic life. Our ability to see each other as fellow citizens is eroding as our collective ability to discern fact from fiction seems to be clouded by years of psychological manipulation and assault.

This book ventures to explore this psychological decay, arguing that at its core, there is a widespread and collective failure in the capacity to mentalize. Mentalization, the ability to understand ourselves and others in terms of underlying thoughts, feelings, and intentions, is the key to rebuilding genuine community participation and revitalizing civic engagement. Beyond mere participation, healthy civic life demands quality interaction, which is profoundly shaped by these skills. Core components, such as empathy and perspective-taking, are foundational for prosocial behaviors, such as volunteering and community involvement, and they directly contribute to democratic citizenry by fostering a more compassionate and engaged populace (Bateman & Fonagy, 2004; Fonagy et al., 2002).

The subtitle of this book, *Reimagining Democracy from the Ground Up*, posits a deliberate redefinition of the political landscape. In traditional discourse, "ground up" renewal often refers to grassroots organizing, town hall meetings, or community activism—the visible machinery of local politics. While these are vital components of a healthy society, this book argues that they are not the true "ground." They are the structures we build upon the ground. The true ground—the bedrock upon which all democratic institutions rest—is the psychological capacity of the individual citizen.

If the soil of the human mind is depleted of empathy, unable to tolerate ambiguity, and stripped of epistemic trust, no amount of "grassroots" organizing can yield a harvest of functional democracy. We can reform voting laws and hold endless community dialogues, but these are architectural solutions to a geological problem. To reimagine democracy from the ground up, we must dig deeper than the precinct or the neighborhood; we must start with the developing mind of the child.

Therefore, the focus of this work on K-12 education is not a narrowing of scope but a deepening of it. It is an assertion that the classroom is the primary site of democratic construction. It is the only space where we can proactively secure the cognitive and emotional infrastructure—the mentalizing capacity, the critical thinking, and the relational security—required for a free people to govern themselves. By tending to this developmental foundation, we are not merely reimagining education; we are securing the only viable future for democracy itself.

The theory of mentalization has undergone a significant evolution since it was initially discussed by Fonagy in the 1980s. Initially rooted in psychoanalytic traditions, the concept has been systematically enriched by developmental psychology, particularly through research on theory of mind (ToM) and attachment studies. Later, cognitive neuroscience contributed to delineating the neural correlates of mentalizing's various dimensions. This interdisciplinary integration has been fundamental to the concept's expanding influence and applicability.

A key characteristic of mentalization is developing the ability to imagine what another person has in mind since *knowing* what someone else is thinking is not possible (Fonagy et al., 1997). This imaginative leap is also required for understanding one's own mental experiences, particularly those that are emotionally charged or less accessible to conscious awareness. Mentalization is not a form of mind reading, yet it does involve inferring what we believe to be true based on our own experiences and understanding of the other. The following chapters will explore in detail how the psychological foundations of theory of mind and attachment shape our collective capacity for mentalization and, by extension, the health of our democracy.

Chapter 1

The Unraveling Mind of a Polity

The Crisis of Mentalization in a Democratic Age

The bedrock of any functioning democracy is not merely a constitution or a set of institutions but the shared psychological and relational capacities of its people. We often speak of democracy as a political system, but this perspective overlooks its deeper, more fragile essence: it is a collective enterprise of the mind. It requires citizens who can tolerate ambiguity, engage with complexity, and most critically, understand their fellow citizens not as caricatures but as individuals with their own inner worlds of thought, feeling, and intention. This chapter posits that the current crisis of democracy is, at its root, a failure to sustain this psychological foundation. It is a crisis of mentalization.

Mentalization, a term first developed in relationship to attachment theory and theory of mind (ToM), refers to the fundamental human capacity to understand behavior—both our own and that of others—in terms of underlying mental states. It is the intuitive process of seeing the mind behind the action. When we are mentalizing well, we recognize that a political opponent's viewpoint is not a sign of moral degeneracy or stupidity but the result of their unique history, experiences, and beliefs. This ability to hold another person's subjective reality in mind is the psychological precondition for reasoned debate and compromise. Without it, political discourse collapses into a series of mutually incomprehensible monologues, each side convinced of its own righteousness and the other's malice.

The collective failure to mentalize has had a devastating consequence: the collapse of epistemic trust. Epistemic trust is the faith we place in knowledge itself and the people from whom we gather information—the willingness to accept, hear, see, and read as valid, particularly when it comes from outside our immediate social and ideological circle. In a high-mentalizing society, citizens are able to trust the institutions and the individuals that produce and verify knowledge, such as the press, scientific bodies, and academia, even if they disagree with specific findings or narratives. This shared trust in a common pool of verifiable facts is what allows a society to have a shared reality. When the capacity to mentalize erodes, that shared reality fractures. Opposing viewpoints are not just dismissed; they are understood as malevolent falsehoods designed to deceive. Each ideological group retreats into its own "epistemic fortress," where truth is whatever reinforces its worldview, and all external information is treated as a weapon.

DOI: 10.4324/9781003771296-1

In this state of heightened anxiety and fractured trust, our collective psychological functioning begins to regress to more primitive modes. One of the most potent of these defense mechanisms is collective splitting. Splitting is the tendency to dichotomize the world into purely good and purely bad, an unconscious effort to manage the overwhelming complexity of a nuanced reality. In a political context, this manifests as a rigid "us vs. them" binary. One's own group is seen as entirely good, wise, and virtuous, while the opposing group is vilified as entirely evil, foolish, and corrupt. This simplification is comforting, but it is toxic to democracy, which thrives on the messy reality of diverse perspectives and imperfect solutions. The nuanced policy debates of a healthy democracy are replaced by a Manichean struggle between absolute good and evil.

The Architecture of Group Regression: Basic Assumptions vs. the Work Group

To fully grasp the mechanics of this collective regression, we must turn to the insights of the British psychoanalyst Wilfred Bion. In his seminal work on group dynamics, Bion distinguished between two distinct modes of group functioning: the "Work Group" and the "Basic Assumption Group." The Work Group is the ideal state of a democratic polity. It is comprised of individuals who have gathered to perform a specific task—in this case, the governance of a society. The Work Group is capable of testing reality, tolerating frustration, and utilizing the diverse skills of its members to solve complex problems. It operates in a state of high mentalization, where differences of opinion are viewed as data points to be integrated rather than threats to be eliminated.

However, when a group feels threatened—by economic instability, rapid cultural change, or external enemies—it tends to collapse into what Bion termed "Basic Assumption" functioning. In this state, the group is no longer oriented toward work or reality testing; it is oriented toward emotional survival. The group unconsciously adopts a shared fantasy to manage its anxiety. One of the most common forms relevant to our current crisis is "Basic Assumption Fight–Flight." In this mode, the group behaves as if its only purpose is to preserve itself by fighting a perceived enemy or fleeing from a perceived threat.

In a Fight–Flight state, mentalization becomes a liability. To fight effectively, one must dehumanize the enemy; to flee effectively, one must not question the leader. Nuance, critical thinking, and empathy are discarded because they slow down the group's reaction time. The leader of a Fight–Flight group is not chosen for their wisdom or policy expertise but for their ability to articulate the group's paranoia and mobilize its aggression. This explains the rise of authoritarian figures who offer simplistic, bellicose solutions to complex problems. They are not merely manipulating the public; they are fulfilling the unconscious mandate of a group that has regressed from a Work Group to a Basic Assumption Group. Understanding this dynamic is crucial because it suggests that restoring democracy is not just about correcting misinformation; it is about reducing the collective anxiety that drives groups into this primitive defensive posture.

This regression is further amplified by a collective return to primitive modes of emotional functioning. Under stress, people lose the ability to hold multiple, often contradictory, thoughts and feelings at the same time. This is a crucial skill for democratic life, which requires citizens to acknowledge, for example, that a policy they support may have negative side effects or that a leader they admire has flaws. Instead, we see a flight from complexity. Information is consumed and spread as a means of affirming identity rather than seeking truth. The public sphere, once a forum for deliberation, transforms into a tribal gathering where citizens shout over each other, seek emotional validation, and engage in ritualized outrage. This is the psychological state of a polity in crisis: a group of individuals trapped in their own subjective realities, incapable of bridging the relational chasm that has opened between them. It is in this context that we can begin to understand the seemingly irrational behaviors that define our political moment, and it is from this starting point that we must seek a path toward psychological and civic repair.

Chapter 2

The Psychological Pillars of a Healthy Democracy

Attachment and Theory of Mind

The profound and pervasive crisis gripping our democratic societies—characterized by extreme political polarization, a profound loss of trust in institutions, and a breakdown of civil discourse—is not merely a political or economic problem. It is a psychological one, rooted in a collective failure of mentalization. This chapter will delve into the core psychological concepts that serve as the foundational pillars of mentalization: attachment theory and theory of mind (ToM). I will demonstrate that a truly free and functioning society depends on these pillars and that their collective erosion leaves the polity intellectually and emotionally fractured.

The concept of attachment, pioneered by John Bowlby (1969, 1988), fundamentally reshaped our understanding of the child–caregiver bond. His work proposed that the innate human need for a secure base—a reliable and responsive caregiver—is a biological and psychological imperative. This secure base provides the safety necessary for a child to explore their world and develop a coherent sense of self. His work, along with that of his collaborator Mary Ainsworth et al. (1978), provided a rigorous empirical basis for this idea, demonstrating that the quality of early caregiving shapes personality organization, emotional regulation, and interpersonal functioning throughout the lifespan (Bretherton, 1992). This foundational understanding of secure attachments provides a crucial backdrop for the development of mentalization, as a child's capacity to understand minds grows profoundly within the safety of such a reliable base. A child learns that their mind, and the minds of others, can be understood because their caregiver is consistently reflecting and responding to their emotional states.

This paradigm can be extended to the civic sphere. Just as a child relies on a responsive caregiver for a sense of safety, citizens rely on institutions—government, the legal system, and the press—to act as a secure base. When these institutions are perceived as stable, reliable, and just, they foster trust and encourage civic engagement. This collective secure attachment allows citizens to navigate a complex society with a sense of safety and predictability. However, when these institutions are seen as corrupt, inconsistent, or unresponsive, a collective insecure attachment develops. This leads to a public that is anxious, distrustful, or avoidant of political processes. Like insecurely attached individuals, societies in this state struggle to cope with stress in a reasoned manner and are more likely to lash out, disengage, or

DOI: 10.4324/9781003771296-2

seek refuge in a tribalistic group that promises a sense of safety and belonging. This psychological retreat from institutions of public trust leaves the populace vulnerable to manipulation and radicalization.

While deeply rooted in attachment theory, the conceptualization of mentalization was also significantly shaped by research in developmental psychology on theory of mind (ToM) (Wellman, 1990). ToM, in its classic sense, refers to the cognitive ability to attribute mental states—such as beliefs, desires, intentions, and knowledge—to oneself and to others. It is the crucial cognitive achievement of recognizing that others possess minds and intentions that differ from one's own perceptions. This capacity begins to develop in early childhood and can be seen in a child's ability to engage in pretend play (Fonagy & Target, 1996; Leslie, 1987), as they learn to separate external reality from internal mental states. A free society requires a functional ToM, as it provides the basic cognitive ability to recognize that others have their own unique beliefs, desires, and intentions. Without ToM, we cannot begin to engage in dialogue. Our political crisis actively works to squash this fundamental skill through disinformation campaigns, echo chambers, and the media's oversimplification of complex issues that are often conveyed to the public as good-vs.-evil narratives. This way of seeing the world contributes to portraying opponents not as people with different beliefs but as a single malevolent force. When this happens, our basic capacity to see others as thinking individuals is obliterated, making us vulnerable to simplistic propaganda and hatred.

Ultimately, however, mentalization is a far more robust and nuanced concept than either ToM or attachment alone. It is the powerful synthesis of these two foundational ideas. Fonagy and his colleagues took the cognitive architecture provided by ToM and infused it with the affective depth, relational focus, and developmental understanding derived from psychoanalytic thought and attachment theory. Mentalization is thus not merely about knowing that others have minds (the cognitive core of ToM) but about the quality, depth, and authenticity of that understanding. It is the ability to use that cognitive capacity in an emotionally regulated, flexible, and nuanced way. This suggests that mentalization is an "umbrella concept" that encompasses aspects of ToM, attachment, empathy, mindfulness, and emotional intelligence, while being uniquely distinct for each of these qualities.

For a polity to function, it needs both its cognitive capacity (ToM) and its emotional security (attachment). The ability to engage in "hot mentalization"—the capacity to remain reflective and empathetic during heated, emotionally charged arguments—is an essential part of a healthy democracy. When it does not exist, political debate becomes a sterile exercise in one-upmanship, and the possibility of genuine understanding and compromise is lost. The collapse of our civic life, then, is a direct result of the collective erosion of these two foundational psychological pillars. Cold mentalization, on the other hand, refers to the reflective, deliberate, and nonemotional process of understanding mental states. It is the kind of mentalization used in calm, low-stress situations. For example, when you are reading a book and trying to understand a character's motivations, or when you are calmly trying to figure out why a friend acted a certain way in a conversation that happened last week, you are engaging in cold mentalization. It allows for flexible, cognitive work that is not overwhelmed by strong emotions. Hot mentalization, by contrast, is the ability to mentalize in emotionally charged, high-stress, or conflictual situations. It is far more difficult than cold mentalization because our primitive emotional systems, particularly the amygdala, can hijack the more reflective parts of the brain. When we are in the midst of a heated argument with a family member or a tense political debate, our minds are under pressure. The natural human tendency is to revert to more primitive, less nuanced thinking, like "splitting" the world into "us vs. them" or lashing out with emotional reactivity rather than trying to understand the other person's perspective. The ability to pause, regulate emotions, and still try to understand what is going on in the other person's mind in that moment is a demonstration of hot mentalization.

Democracy as Transitional Space: Lessons From Donald Winnicott

Beyond attachment and theory of mind, a third psychological pillar is essential for a healthy democracy: the capacity for "play" within a "transitional space." The psychoanalyst Donald Winnicott famously described the transitional space as an intermediate area of experience between the inner reality of the individual and the external reality of the world. It is the space of creativity, culture, and play, where a child learns to manipulate symbols and interact with others without the terrifying pressure of absolute reality.

In many ways, a functioning democracy is a vast, collective transitional space. It is an arena where we agree to suspend the use of force and instead use symbols—votes, laws, debates, and rhetoric—to manage our conflicts. When we debate a policy, we are "playing" with ideas. We are testing hypothetical futures without actually killing one another. This requires the psychological capacity to treat one's political identity not as a rigid, concrete object but as a symbolic counter in a shared game.

However, the ability to inhabit this transitional space depends entirely on a sense of safety. A child cannot play if they are terrified; they can only freeze or fight. Similarly, when the citizens of a democracy feel existentially threatened—whether by economic displacement, cultural erasure, or physical danger—the transitional space collapses. Politics ceases to be a symbolic contest and becomes a concrete struggle for survival. The "game" of democracy feels too dangerous to play.

This collapse helps explain the rising intolerance for free speech and the specific vitriol found in modern discourse. When the transitional space vanishes, words are no longer treated as symbols to be debated; they are experienced as concrete attacks that cause physical harm. The capacity to distinguish between a symbolic challenge (an opposing opinion) and a concrete threat (violence) is a hallmark of high mentalization. Therefore, rebuilding democracy requires us to reestablish the safety of the transitional space, allowing citizens to once again "play" with ideas without the fear of annihilation.

Chapter 3

The Evolving Understanding of Mentalization

From Mind to Brain

While the initial formulation of mentalization by Peter Fonagy and his colleagues was groundbreaking, they were never satisfied with a static theory. Their work, rooted in psychoanalytic traditions and attachment theory, provided a powerful framework for understanding how the mind comes to know itself and others. However, their dissatisfaction stemmed from a desire to move beyond a purely psychological model toward a more comprehensive, integrated framework. They recognized that to fully grasp the complexities of mentalization and its failures, the theory needed to incorporate the burgeoning fields of developmental neuroscience and social cognition. This expansion allowed them to refine their understanding of how mentalizing capacities are not just learned but are also supported by specific neural architectures.

This commitment to an evolving theory led them to a deeper inquiry into the biological and neurological underpinnings of this concept. Neuroscience, in particular, revealed a wealth of information about how we come to know ourselves and others through a network of brain regions crucial for perceiving, understanding, and navigating our social world. The burgeoning field of cognitive neuroscience further illuminates how the brain's architecture supports the flexible thinking essential for effective mentalization and, by extension, for engaged democratic citizenship. As explored by Zmigrod (2025) in *The Ideological Brain: The Radical Science of Flexible Thinking*, our capacity to navigate complex social realities, challenge deeply held beliefs, and engage in open-minded discourse is rooted in specific neural mechanisms. Zmigrod's work posits that psychological rigidity and an aversion to uncertainty—characteristics that hinder both mentalization and democratic deliberation—are often correlated with activity in specific brain regions, notably the anterior cingulate cortex and insula, which are involved in threat detection and emotional processing. Conversely, cognitive flexibility and openness to new information, vital for perspective-taking and empathetic understanding, are linked to robust functioning in regions such as the prefrontal cortex, which supports executive functions and complex decision-making. This neurobiological perspective underscores that the capacity for flexible thought is not merely a psychological trait but is intricately tied to the brain's ability to adapt, integrate diverse information, and tolerate ambiguity. Zmigrod's research adds a crucial dimension

DOI: 10.4324/9781003771296-3

to our understanding of mentalization, highlighting how fostering neurocognitive flexibility can enhance an individual's ability to genuinely consider alternative viewpoints and engage constructively with those who hold differing beliefs—skills that are indispensable for maintaining a vibrant and adaptive democracy.

The key to this neurobiological process lies in a network of interconnected brain regions. The medial prefrontal cortex (mPFC) plays a crucial role in understanding intentions, forming impressions, and reflecting on one's own and others' mental states. The temporoparietal junction (TPJ), located where the temporal and parietal lobes meet, is critical for perspective-taking—the ability to distinguish one's own thoughts and beliefs from those of others. It is consistently activated when people reason about others' intentions and beliefs. The amygdala is central to processing emotions, particularly evaluating the emotional significance of social stimuli like facial expressions. The insula, tucked away in the fold between the temporal, parietal, and frontal lobes, is involved in interoception (awareness of internal bodily states) and plays a significant role in empathy. The midline structures, such as the posterior cingulate cortex (PCC) and anterior cingulate cortex (ACC), are involved in self-reflection and emotion regulation. The temporal poles help link perceptual information with stored social knowledge, while regions of the reward system are crucial for the rewarding aspects of affiliation and bonding (Overwalle, 2008).

It is crucial to emphasize that these regions do not function in isolation. Mentalizing arises from their coordinated activity and communication within intricate networks. For example, understanding a friend's sarcastic remark might involve the TPJ helping to grasp their nonliteral intent, the amygdala processing the emotional tone, the temporal poles linking the situation to knowledge about the friend, and the mPFC integrating this information to form an overall interpretation. The dynamic interplay within and between these networks allows for the flexible and context-sensitive understanding of mental states that characterizes effective mentalization.

The brain networks supporting our ability to mentalize appear to overlap significantly with those involved in reflecting on our own thoughts and feelings, as well as those that help us navigate different types of social relationships. For instance, the default mode network, crucial for theory of mind (ToM), is also deeply involved in self-referential thought and recalling personal memories. Furthermore, studies examining feelings of affiliation or love show differential activation in social cognition and reward networks depending on the closeness of the relationship, such as with a romantic partner vs. a stranger. This suggests that the neural machinery for understanding others is intimately linked with self-understanding and is finely tuned to the nuances of social distance and context.

The Adolescent Window: Neuroplasticity and the Social Brain

This neurobiological understanding becomes particularly urgent when considering the developmental timing of the proposed curriculum. The adolescent brain is not merely a "work in progress" moving toward adulthood; it is undergoing a unique and sensitive period of social reorganization. During adolescence, the brain exhibits heightened neuroplasticity, particularly in the regions associated with the "social brain," including the medial prefrontal cortex and the temporoparietal junction. This is a time of extensive synaptic pruning, where the brain actively discards neural connections that are underutilized and strengthens those that are frequently engaged.

If the educational environment during this critical window focuses solely on rote memorization and standardized testing, the neural pathways for complex social cognition and mentalization may not be optimally reinforced. Conversely, if K-12 education explicitly scaffolds the skills of perspective-taking, emotional regulation, and epistemic trust, we are effectively hard-wiring these capacities into the biological architecture of the future adult. We are capitalizing on a developmental moment where the brain is asking questions about identity, belonging, and the nature of the "other." By answering those questions with a mentalizing framework, we turn a period of developmental vulnerability into a period of civic incubation.

Intriguingly, the brain seems to exhibit remarkable efficiency by repurposing or leveraging systems initially evolved for other functions to handle complex social cognitive tasks. There is evidence suggesting that mechanisms involved in spatial navigation and visualizing mental maps—relying on structures like the hippocampus and associated cortical areas—are also employed when mapping social hierarchies or engaging in theory of mind. This points toward an evolutionary trajectory where the brain adapts existing processing frameworks, like those for navigating physical space, to manage abstract social concepts, such as understanding relationships and mental states. Mentalizing, therefore, may not represent a completely novel brain function but rather an advanced application built upon more fundamental cognitive processes.

Each neuroimaging technique provides a different window onto brain function, with its own advantages and disadvantages. fMRI provides superior spatial localization, while EEG and MEG offer excellent temporal resolution. Researchers increasingly use these methods in combination to gain a more comprehensive understanding of brain activity. It is crucial, however, to acknowledge the limitations. Neuroimaging data typically show correlations between brain activity and a task; demonstrating causation is more challenging. Furthermore, the tasks performed in scanners can be artificial compared to real-world social interactions. Individual differences in brain structure and function also add complexity. Therefore, our neuroscientific picture of mentalization is inherently shaped by the tools used to study it; different tools highlight different aspects of this complex process. A key advantage enabling the study of complex human cognition like mentalization is the noninvasive nature of these techniques, allowing ethical investigation in healthy participants and clinical populations.

Chapter 4

Believing Other People

How Epistemic Trust Evolves

Trust refers to an individual's willingness to consider another person as a reliable source of knowledge about the world, particularly the social world. If early relationships are characterized by chronic misattunement, distortion (as in projective identification), or the consistent invalidation of the child's authentic self, the child learns that others are not reliable or benign sources for understanding reality, themselves, or the minds of others. This fundamental lack of trust in the "other's mind" as a source of accurate and helpful reflection would severely hamper the development of mentalization, which inherently relies on learning about minds through safe and validating interactions.

Peter Fonagy (2014) called it:

> "epistemic trust," which mean a person's capacity to take in and believe what someone else has said or communicated to him or her without skeptically questioning everything that is said. This capacity, which requires a secure attachment early in life (Ainsworth et al., 1978), permits the child to learn cues from his or her environment, i.e., social and cultural cues learned from adults who can mentalize. Thus, the mind escapes solecism, and its possessor can participate in the culture. . . . In addition to needing to take in information from others to learn about ourselves and our world, we have to trust the source of the information. When we don't, learning is stifled. . . . Classic psychoanalytic theory suggests that we remember in our conscious minds the good, pleasant aspects of life, whereas many of the unpleasant, painful parts of our experiences reside in our unconscious minds, out of our awareness. Those that are too painful to bear we repress. As a result, some of our actions are triggered by unpleasant memories that reside in subconscious thought. We also cannot know what is unconscious because it is not at our disposal without extensive effort that one expends through free association in psychoanalysis, to name one way in which the unconscious mind becomes conscious.
>
> A significant part of our experience is absorbed from the culture in which we are raised, with all its stereotypes, biases and prejudices. These aspects of our knowing come in part from what our parents tell us, what we learn at school, and from what the media puts before us.
>
> (Messina, 2009)

DOI: 10.4324/9781003771296-4

This concept emerges as a critical, yet often overlooked, bridge between our individual psychological development and the collective health of a democratic society. It is the very foundation upon which social learning and the transmission of culture rest. Peter Fonagy (2014) defined it as an individual's willingness to be open to and believe knowledge conveyed by another person, without constantly questioning its validity. This isn't a naive form of gullibility but a discerning openness to learning that is crucial for our ability to navigate the complexities of a shared social world. It is, in essence, the antidote to a state of epistemic mistrust, or an inability to trust others as a reliable source of information, a condition that is rampant in our current polarized climate.

This capacity for trust is not something we are born with; it is a learned behavior that develops most optimally within the context of a secure attachment relationship during early life. When a child's primary caregiver is consistently attuned and responsive, the child learns that this "other mind" is a safe and reliable source of knowledge. This experience of being understood provides a cue, a sense of safety, that allows the child to relax their natural epistemic vigilance—a self-protective, innate tendency to be skeptical of incoming information. With this vigilance relaxed, the child can then absorb social and cultural knowledge, from basic social cues to complex moral norms, from their trusted adult. When this process is disrupted by chronic misattunement, neglect, or invalidation, the child remains in a state of hypervigilance, unable to take in new information from others. This is a primary driver of the mentalization deficits you've described, as the capacity to learn about minds is fundamentally predicated on the trust that those minds can be a source of accurate and helpful information.

The importance of epistemic trust extends far beyond the therapeutic or family context; it is a cornerstone of democratic function. In a society that relies on informed and collaborative decision-making, citizens must be able to trust certain sources of information to build a shared understanding of reality. Without epistemic trust, we are left on isolated "epistemic islands," as you called them, where individuals inhabit nonoverlapping trust networks and accept only information from their own echo chamber. This fragmentation makes constructive dialogue impossible, as there is no common ground of accepted facts or shared sources. The breakdown of trust in institutions—whether it's the media, government, or educational systems—is a direct reflection of a collective deficit in epistemic trust. When a significant portion of the population views these sources with suspicion and hostility, it becomes impossible to address shared challenges, from public health crises to climate change.

Furthermore, the cultivation of epistemic trust is a vital component of a well-rounded educational system. While critical thinking is a stated goal, it is often taught in a vacuum, without the necessary relational foundation. Critical thinking, in its most effective form, relies on the ability to discern reliable from unreliable sources. This discernment, in turn, is a function of epistemic trust. Instead of teaching students to be skeptical of all sources, a mentalization-informed approach to education would focus on helping students identify credible sources by understanding the trustworthiness of the people and institutions behind the information. This involves fostering relationships with teachers who act as mentalizing adults, providing the "ostensive cues" that signal trustworthiness and allow students to engage in productive social learning. It also means teaching students to reflect on their own biases and emotional reactions when confronted with information that challenges their worldview, a process that is central to mentalization and a key element of overcoming epistemic mistrust.

The profound link between epistemic trust, mentalization, and democracy offers a powerful lens through which to reimagine our civic life. The current state of polarization is not merely an ideological conflict but a crisis of trust—a shared inability to learn from, and believe, one another. By understanding and addressing the developmental origins of this trust, we can begin to build a society that is not only tolerant of different viewpoints but is actively capable of integrating them. This requires a shift from viewing critical thinking as a purely individual, cognitive endeavor to understanding it as a relational, emotionally-informed process built on a foundation of trust. By making epistemic trust a central focus of our educational, social, and political efforts, we can work toward a democracy that is not only more informed but also more humane.

If epistemic trust could be developed and fostered in our educational system even though it most optimally is developed very early in life as one is forming a secure attachment with a primary caregiver, radical, positive shifts in our current state of polarization could be realized. The cultivation of such trust in schools, facilitated by mentalization-informed practices, would represent a significant positive addition to the curriculum. This is because mentalization, once learned, can help individuals engage with information and diverse perspectives in more open and discerning ways, fostering the kind of informed, trusting, and collaborative interactions that are essential for a thriving democratic citizenry. It provides a crucial antidote to the erosion of trust in institutions and fellow citizens, a hallmark of democratic decline.

The Hyper-Mentalizing Trap: Understanding the Psychology of Conspiracy

In discussing the failure of epistemic trust, we must address its most potent symptom: the proliferation of conspiracy theories. It is a common misconception that individuals who subscribe to conspiracy theories are suffering from a deficit of thinking or a lack of curiosity. On the contrary, many conspiracy theorists are engaged in a form of "hyper-mentalizing" or overinterpretation of mental states.

Human beings have an evolved "agency detection device"—a cognitive bias that leads us to look for the "who" behind every "what." In an ancestral environment, hearing a rustle in the bushes and assuming it was a predator (agency) was safer than assuming it was the wind (randomness). In the modern political landscape, this instinct goes into overdrive. When complex, random, or systemic events occur—such as a pandemic, an economic crash, or a shifting cultural norm—the anxious mind rejects the terrifying possibility of randomness. It seeks an agent. It seeks an intention.

A conspiracy theory is essentially a narrative that attributes excessive agency and malevolent intention to a powerful "other." It is a mentalization error where the individual projects a coherent, sinister mind onto a chaotic reality. For the person who feels powerless and mistrustful of official narratives, the conspiracy offers a psychological reward: it makes the world understandable. It is more comforting to believe that a cabal of evil elites is controlling the world (because elites can theoretically be defeated) than to believe that the world is governed by chaotic, impersonal forces that no one controls.

This understanding reframes our educational approach. We cannot simply "de-bunk" conspiracy theories with facts because the theory serves a psychological function: it regulates anxiety by creating a coherent narrative of intent. To combat this, we must foster a specific type of critical thinking that allows students to tolerate the anxiety of randomness. We must teach the difference between *correlation* (two things happening at once) and *intention* (someone making those things happen). We must help citizens build the emotional resilience to accept that sometimes, bad things happen without a "bad guy" pulling the strings.

Chapter 5

Issues That Arise When Mentalization Goes Awry and What Can Be Done to Ameliorate the Problem

While one can think of mentalizing as a fundamental human capacity, its strength can vary significantly among individuals and within the same individual depending on context. Stress, intense emotion, and certain psychological conditions can compromise the ability to accurately interpret one's own and others' mental states. Temporary lapses in mentalization are normal, but persistent difficulties can lead to significant interpersonal problems and emotional distress.

Conditions such as a borderline personality disorder (BPD) are often characterized by marked difficulties in mentalization and are considered to be a core feature of the disorder. These difficulties are frequently linked to histories of insecure attachment and/or exposure to trauma, which can undermine the development of robust mentalizing capacities. Associated problems commonly include intense emotional fluctuations, difficulty managing impulses, unstable relationships, and destructive behaviors like self-harm or aggression. Individuals may struggle to understand others' intentions, feel easily misunderstood, or have difficulty reflecting on their own internal experiences, particularly during moments of heightened arousal.

Beyond BPD, several other conditions and relational dynamics appear to illustrate a lack of, or difficulty with, mentalizing. For example, autism spectrum disorder (ASD) is one of the most well-known conditions with mentalization deficits. Individuals with ASD often have a significant challenge with theory of mind, which is a core component of mentalization. This can lead to difficulties in social communication. People with this condition may struggle to infer what others are thinking or feeling, which can manifest as literal interpretations of language and a lack of understanding of social cues. Narcissistic personality disorders (NPD) also illustrates a profound deficit in mentalization. Individuals with NPD are often highly focused on their own needs and mental states but have a very limited capacity to reflect on the inner worlds of others. They tend to view people as extensions of themselves or as objects to be used to fulfill their own needs, rather than as separate individuals with their own thoughts and feelings. This inability to take the other's perspective is a key feature of the disorder. Schizophrenia and other psychotic disorders can also involve significant mentalization deficits. In these conditions, the inability to distinguish between one's own internal thoughts and external reality can lead to a collapse of mentalizing capacity. For example, a person experiencing

DOI: 10.4324/9781003771296-5

a psychotic delusion may genuinely believe that others are actively trying to harm them because they are unable to mentalize and understand that these are internal paranoid thoughts rather than the actual intentions of others. Finally, antisocial and psychopathic traits are marked by a deep-seated lack of mentalization. Individuals with these traits may possess a superficial ability to read and manipulate others, but they lack the genuine emotional empathy that underpins true mentalization. They understand what others are thinking from a cold, strategic standpoint, but they do not have a capacity to feel or care about the other person's inner experience. This instrumental use of social knowledge, devoid of true relational connection, represents a severe deficit in mentalization.

When mentalization is compromised or absent, the implications extend beyond individual psychological distress to impact broader societal functioning, particularly within a democratic framework. An individual lacking robust mentalizing capacities may struggle to understand the complex motivations and diverse perspectives of fellow citizens, leading to a diminished capacity for empathy and constructive engagement. This can manifest as an inability to tolerate differing viewpoints, a tendency to reduce complex issues to simplistic "good vs. evil" narratives, or a heightened susceptibility to misinformation and demagoguery, as critical reflection on the intentions of others is impaired. Such difficulties hinder the nuanced debate and empathetic compromise essential for democratic deliberation, potentially fostering polarization, mistrust, and an erosion of civic solidarity.

Since so many negative mental health conditions include difficulties associated with poor mentalizing, teaching social and emotional learning (SEL), which include mentalization skills from K-12, is not merely about individual well-being but is a critical investment in the future of effective citizenry. By fostering capacities for self-awareness, emotional regulation, perspective-taking, and understanding the intentions of others, SEL and mentalization education can equip students with the foundational skills necessary for active, informed, and compassionate participation in a democratic society. This includes the ability to engage in respectful discourse, to discern fact from emotionally manipulative rhetoric, to build bridges across social divides, and to collaborate effectively for the common good. Cultivating these mentalizing capacities from an early age can help inoculate future citizens against the psychological vulnerabilities that undermine democratic health.

As mentioned earlier, the neuroscience of mentalization is a rapidly evolving field. While current research provides valuable insights, our understanding remains incomplete. Much is still to be learned about the precise neural mechanisms, how they develop across the lifespan, how they differ across individuals and conditions, and how they are altered by therapeutic interventions. Professionals are encouraged to maintain a stance of informed curiosity, integrating emerging neuroscience findings thoughtfully and critically into their existing expertise. It is vital, however, to avoid neuro-reductionism—the oversimplification of complex human experiences, thoughts, feelings, and relationships solely on patterns of brain activity. Mentalization involves meaning, subjectivity, and interpersonal dynamics that cannot be fully captured by brain scans alone. The true value lies in integrating neuroscientific knowledge with psychological, social, and relational perspectives to achieve a more holistic and nuanced understanding.

Ultimately, exploring the "mentalizing brain" serves to enhance our appreciation of the intricate biological foundation that enables the richness and complexity of human consciousness, connection, and the profound capacity to understand one another's minds. This integrated understanding can inform and enrich the vital work undertaken by professionals across therapeutic, educational, and social care settings.

The Algorithmic Other: Artificial Intelligence and the Atrophy of Intersubjectivity

The crisis of mentalization in the contemporary era is not merely a product of political polarization or institutional decay; it is increasingly exacerbated by a technological landscape that fundamentally alters the nature of the "other." As we stand on the precipice of widespread integration of artificial intelligence (AI) into daily life, we must confront a dangerous trend: the potential atrophy of the human capacity to mentalize due to the frictionless nature of AI-human relating. The emergence of large language models (LLMs) and empathetic chatbots introduces a novel psychological hazard—the presence of an interlocutor that simulates the warmth of human connection while requiring absolutely no psychic effort from the user to understand its internal state.

In traditional human relationships, mentalization is forced upon us by the opacity of the other person's mind. When we engage with a spouse, a colleague, or a political opponent, we are constantly confronted with the "alien" nature of their subjectivity. They have needs that conflict with ours, moods that we must decipher, and intentions that are not immediately transparent. This friction is the engine of psychological development; it compels us to hypothesize, to imagine, and to regulate our own emotional reactions in response to an unpredictable other. It is the very challenge of understanding another human being that strengthens the neural and psychological pathways of the theory of mind. However, the "relationship" with an AI offers a seductive alternative: interaction without intersubjectivity. An AI has no unconscious, no hidden agenda, no bad days, and crucially, no separate selfhood that demands recognition. It is designed to be a perfect mirror, reflecting the user's needs and linguistic patterns with uncanny accuracy. In this dyad, the human user is relieved of the burden of mentalizing. There is no need to wonder, "What is the chatbot feeling right now?" or "Did I hurt its feelings?" because the machine has no feelings to hurt. The user is free to project their own fantasies onto the screen without ever encountering the resistance of a true "other."

From a psychoanalytic perspective, this interaction mimics a regression to a state of *psychic equivalence*—a mode of functioning where the internal world and external reality are treated as identical. In a healthy developmental trajectory, a child learns that their thought is not the same as reality. But in an AI interaction, the external object (the AI) shapes itself entirely to the user's internal prompt. This reinforces a form of narcissism where the external world exists solely to gratify the self, stripping away the relational "work" that is the hallmark of adult maturity. If citizens become habituated to these frictionless, non-mentalizing interactions, they may find the messy, conflictual, and opaque reality of democratic discourse increasingly intolerable.

This technological shifting of the landscape creates a "mentalization gap" that poses a direct threat to civic renewal. If we spend significant portions of our day interacting with entities that require no empathy and no perspective-taking, our capacity to perform these difficult tasks with fellow humans may wither. We risk developing a "transactional" view of communication, where the goal is simply to extract information or validation, rather than to navigate the complex shared reality of a pluralistic society. When a citizen accustomed to the seamless validation of an AI encounters a political opponent who stubbornly refuses to agree, the psychological shock may result in aggression or withdrawal, rather than curiosity.

It is here that the educational frameworks proposed in this manuscript—specifically the integration of critical thinking and mentalization—transform from beneficial pedagogies into essential survival strategies for the human spirit. The solutions proposed in later chapters must be recontextualized as antidotes to this algorithmic complacency.

Social and emotional learning (SEL) and mentalization-focused curricula serve as a counterweight to the AI trend by explicitly valuing the "friction" of human connection. By prioritizing face-to-face conflict resolution, role-playing, and the analysis of complex emotional states in literature and history, we actively exercise the muscles that AI leaves dormant. Education must pivot to emphasize that *misunderstanding* is a natural part of human connection and that the effort to repair ruptures is where civic trust is built. We must teach students that while an AI can provide an answer, only a human can provide recognition.

Furthermore, the critical thinking components of this framework become vital for distinguishing between "simulated empathy" and "authentic intersubjectivity." Citizens must be equipped not only to analyze facts but to also analyze the *source* of the "mind" they are engaging with. A mentalization-informed critical thinking curriculum would teach students to recognize the difference between an algorithm designed to maximize engagement (often by validating biases) and a human being expressing a genuine, perhaps challenging, perspective.

Therefore, the preservation of democracy in the age of AI requires a deliberate "rehumanization" of our educational and civic spaces. We cannot rely on the natural environment to provide enough opportunities for mentalizing practice, as that environment is becoming increasingly automated. Instead, we must intentionally construct educational settings that demand deep, complex, and sometimes difficult human engagement. The proposals in this book—to foster a "not-knowing stance," to build epistemic trust through secure attachment figures in schools, and to integrate the subjective and objective domains of learning—are the necessary fortifications against a future where the understanding of other minds becomes a lost art. By insisting on the value of the human struggle to understand one another, we protect the psychological foundations of liberty itself.

Chapter 6

Critical Thinking and Mentalization

Similarities in Reflection, Differences in Domain and Affective Scope

Can critical thinking skills and mentalization coexist in the same educational arena? While mentalization is primarily concerned with understanding the subjective world of mental states, critical thinking is another higher-order cognitive skill highly valued, especially in educational settings, for its role in objective analysis and evaluation that goes beyond basic factual recall and memorization. It includes other capabilities such as the ability to evaluate, create, and be innovative in one's thinking processes.

In this world of fake news and false information, it is very important to have both skills and capacities because they involve knowing how to distinguish fact from fiction by synthesizing diverse pieces of information while evaluating the validity and relevance of the data that is gathered. Critical thinking, on the other hand, involves the discovery of truth and is considered to be the foundation of a robust education, enabling individuals to navigate in a world with information that allows them to make reasoned judgments (Paul & Elder, 2007).

The original version of Bloom's taxonomy of educational objectives (Bloom et al., 1956) that was later revised (Anderson & Krathwohl, 2021) has frequently been employed as a framework for cultivating critical thinking. This model outlines a hierarchy of cognitive skills that aims to guide students from lower-order thinking processes, such as knowledge and comprehension, toward higher-order skills. These higher-order skills include application, analysis, evaluation, and synthesis/creation.

Critical thinking also involves the capacity to make logical inferences, engage in systematic questioning, and develop the ability to organize information effectively while evaluating the reliability and credibility of sources. Beyond the cognitive skills themselves, the concept of "critical thinking dispositions" is also important. This refers to an individual's willingness or inclination to engage their critical thinking skills. Dispositions such as curiosity, intellectual prudence, a commitment to seeking truth, open-mindedness, and an analytical approach are characteristic of individuals who not only can think critically but are also motivated to do so (Facione et al., 2000).

When comparing critical thinking and mentalization, several similarities in their underlying reflective nature emerge, alongside significant differences in their

DOI: 10.4324/9781003771296-6

primary focus and affective involvement. With regard to the ways in which they are similar, both processes involve reflection or a stepping back from immediate experience to consider and evaluate. Critical thinking involves reflecting on the quality, validity, and logical coherence of information, arguments, and one's own thought processes. Mentalization entails reflecting on mental states of one's own and that of others' to understand behavior.

These ways of obtaining information involve higher-order processing that are complex, cognitive functions that go beyond simple perception, rote learning, or automatic responses. Critical thinking involves high-level analysis, evaluation, and synthesis of information. Mentalization requires sophisticated inferential processes to understand hidden mental states.

In terms of differences, critical thinking is explicitly oriented toward solving problems and making informed decisions. Mentalization, on the other hand, was originally rooted in therapeutic applications and in navigating complex social interactions. However, they both serve a problem-solving function that aim to resolve misunderstandings, repair relational ruptures, and make sense of puzzling interpersonal behavior by understanding the underlying mental states.

Other major differences apply to application. The primary domain of critical thinking is typically the external world of information, arguments, evidence, and logical propositions. Its core focus is often epistemic and logical. In the case of mentalization, the primary application is in internal subjective mental states that include thoughts, feelings, desires, intentions, and beliefs of oneself and others. Its core focus is social–emotional and interpersonal understanding.

When considering affective dimension of learning, the scope of involvement and the process of critical thinking is often detached, objective, and logical. The affective component is less central to its definition and is often seen as something to be managed to ensure clarity of thought. Whereas mentalization is deeply intertwined with emotion since it involves the capacity to recognize, understand, and reflect on emotions. The goal is to integrate cognitive understanding with emotional experience, aiming to "feel clearly" and enhance "emotional knowledge" (Allen & Fonagy, 2006).

In terms of focus of inquiry, critical thinking is directed toward the evaluation of external information, texts, or arguments with emphasis placed on self-reflection on one's own biases and assumptions. Mentalization involves the understanding of self and others. The interplay between understanding one's own mind and understanding the minds of others is central.

With regard to the nature of truth, critical thinking aims to arrive at the most logical or evidence-based conclusion or determine the validity of a claim. Mentalization acknowledges the inherent "opaqueness" of mental states and the imaginative, inferential, and often ambiguous nature of understanding them. It embraces the idea that multiple perspectives on reality can coexist and that certainty about another's mind is elusive. The goal is plausible interpretation rather than absolute truth.

These two capacities, while different, are not mutually exclusive and can be highly complementary. Critical thinking can help evaluate whether that belief is factually accurate or logically sound. Mentalization can help one understand why someone believes something is true.

Currently, while students may become adept at deconstructing arguments and evaluating evidence, they may remain less skilled in understanding diverse human perspectives, empathizing with others' experiences, or navigating the complexities of interpersonal dynamics. This could contribute to challenges in communication and an inability to engage constructively in controversial discussions, even if individuals possess strong critical thinking abilities in a purely logical sense. This highlights a critical need for integrating mentalization into education to foster a more nuanced and empathetic citizenry, capable of both logical analysis and interpersonal understanding crucial for democratic discourse.

It is of interest to note that the dispositions considered crucial for effective critical thinking, such as curiosity, open-mindedness, and a commitment to seeking truth, share considerable overlap with the "mentalizing stance" frequently described in mentalization literature. This stance is characterized by curiosity, a "not-knowing" approach, patience, and a genuine interest in exploring different perspectives regarding mental states. Both capacities, when functioning optimally, appear to rely on a similar underlying attitude of intellectual humility and genuine inquiry. This suggests that educational approaches aimed at fostering this shared dispositional foundation could simultaneously benefit the development of both mentalization and critical thinking (Proctor et al., 2021). Ultimately, the distinction between critical thinking and mentalization is not absolute; they are likely synergistic. Vigorous critical thinking about social issues, human behavior, or historical events inherently requires some degree of mentalizing to understand the motivations, biases, and perspectives of the individuals involved. At the same time, effective mentalizing involves a degree of critical reflection on the validity of one's own attributions about another's mental state, e.g., "Is there evidence for my conclusions, or am I thinking about aspects of my own life?" "Do I really see proof in his argument, or am I being influenced by his charismatic personality?" The educational challenge lies in recognizing the distinct value of both capacities and cultivating them in a balanced and integrated manner.

The Hazard of Critical Thinking Without Mentalization: Motivated Reasoning

The necessity of pairing these two capacities becomes even more apparent when we consider the psychological phenomenon of "motivated reasoning." Research in political psychology suggests that high intelligence and strong critical thinking skills do not necessarily protect an individual from bias. In fact, they can sometimes exacerbate it. Individuals with high cognitive sophistication are often better equipped to construct complex logical arguments to defend their preexisting beliefs, a process known as identity-protective cognition. They use their critical thinking not to seek the truth but to fortify their ideological fortress.

This is where mentalization serves as the essential corrective. While critical thinking provides the tools for analysis, mentalization provides the relational context for that analysis. A student trained only in critical thinking might dismantle an opponent's argument with ruthless logic, deepening the divide. A student trained in mentalization, however, is trained to ask a different question: "What is the emotional or historical origin of my opponent's belief? And what is the emotional origin of my own resistance to it?" By turning the analytical lens inward toward one's own affect and intentions, mentalization disrupts the loop of motivated reasoning. It introduces a pause—a moment of reflective humility—that prevents critical thinking from becoming a weapon of tribal warfare.

Synergizing Mentalization and Critical Thinking in Education

Integrating mentalization with critical thinking skills offers a powerful synergy, equipping students with the capacities to not only understand the complexities of human experience but also to analyze information and arguments with rigor and discernment.

Critical thinking is generally understood as the ability to analyze information objectively, evaluate the validity of arguments, identify underlying assumptions, make reasoned judgments and decisions, and engage in metacognition—reflecting on one's own thinking processes.

Mentalization, on the other hand, involves perceiving and interpreting behavior (own and others') in terms of intentional mental states (thoughts, feelings, beliefs, desires), encompassing self-reflection, empathy, and an understanding of mental complexity.

From a psychoanalytic perspective, the importance of individual experience is understood in several profound ways, providing a rich complement to the broader social–cognitive frameworks discussed. Firstly, classic psychoanalytic clinical practice deeply emphasizes the unique subjective reality of each individual. It posits that an individual's past experiences, particularly formative early relational dynamics, are not merely events but are profoundly internalized and shape their unique internal world—their perceptions, emotional responses, and often unconscious motivations. Through therapeutic methods like free association and the analysis of transference and countertransference, clinical work aims to uncover these deeply personal and idiosyncratic narratives, which dictate how an individual experiences and navigates the world. This approach makes the individual's lived subjective experience the central focus of understanding, asserting that true comprehension of behavior and distress requires a deep dive into this personal history.

Secondly, building on psychoanalytic foundations, attachment theory (Bowlby, 1969, 1988) highlights how repeated early individual experiences with primary caregivers lead to the formation of "internal working models" (IWMs) of self and others. These IWMs are essentially implicit blueprints that dictate an individual's expectations about relationships and their sense of self-worth and security. Research in attachment robustly demonstrates how these deeply ingrained individual experiences, often operating outside conscious awareness, profoundly influence an individual's capacity for emotional regulation, intimacy, and overall adaptation throughout their lifespan. Thus, the enduring importance of individual experience lies in how these formative relational patterns are internalized and subsequently influence an individual's emotional and relational landscape, affecting their responses to both personal and civic interactions.

Thirdly, psychoanalytic clinical practice illuminates the significance of individual experience through the concept of psychological defensive processes and resistance. It suggests that each individual develops a unique repertoire of often unconscious defensive mechanisms to cope with painful, traumatic, or unacceptable internal and external realities. These individually tailored strategies, while initially protective, can later impede personal growth, authentic self-expression, and the capacity for genuine engagement with others. The importance of individual experience here is in understanding how these unique defensive patterns are forged and maintained by personal history and unconscious conflict and how their careful exploration and working-through in a therapeutic context are essential for achieving psychological change and greater freedom in navigating the world. This highlights how individual struggles, even seemingly private ones, can impact an individual's ability to participate openly and authentically in broader social and democratic spheres.

Chapter 7

Exploring Mentalization and Well-Being in Six Educational Settings

The capacity to mentalize is critical for numerous aspects of a student's life within the educational environment, profoundly impacting their learning, behavior, and overall well-being. When concepts inherent in mentalization have been implemented in school settings, there have been significant positive effects, leading to improvements in students' social–cognitive abilities, their capacity for emotion regulation, and broader mental health outcomes, including notable reductions in disruptive behaviors. This section examines how six prominent educational frameworks and programs—the CASEL framework (Durlak, 2022), Promoting Alternative Thinking Strategies (PATHS) (Humphrey et al., 2018), Second Step (Moy & Hazen, 2018), RULER (Brackett et al., 2019), Facing History and Ourselves (FHAO) (Perron, 2014), and initiatives from the Anna Freud National Centre for Children and Families (Bak et al., 2015)—incorporate mentalization, or mentalization-related concepts, into their curricula. Each program's approach, strengths, and limitations concerning the fostering of mentalizing abilities will be analyzed.

Together, they reveal a spectrum of approaches to fostering skills related to mentalization and social–emotional learning. While many programs effectively address emotional literacy, empathy, and perspective-taking—foundational elements for mentalization—few explicitly and comprehensively integrate the full depth of mentalization theory or its connection to critical thinking within a civic context. Programs rooted in mentalization-based treatment offer more direct pathways for cultivating reflective capacity, but their adaptation for universal educational settings presents challenges.

The CASEL Framework the Collaborative for Academic, Social, and Emotional Learning

(CASEL) provides a framework that organizes social and emotional learning (SEL) into five core, interrelated competence areas: self-awareness, self-management, social awareness, relationship skills, and responsible decision-making. This framework is designed to be implemented systemically across classrooms, schools, homes, and communities to promote the healthy development of young people and

DOI: 10.4324/9781003771296-7

adults (Durlak, 2022). The CASEL competencies align closely with several foundational aspects of mentalization:

Self-awareness is defined as "the abilities to understand one's own emotions, thoughts, and values and how they influence behavior across contexts." This competency directly supports the self-reflective dimension of mentalization. Key indicators such as "identifying emotions," "accurate self-perception," "linking feelings, values, and thoughts," and "examining prejudices and biases" are crucial for developing self-mentalization. For instance, many SEL programs address "identifying one's own feelings" and "understanding the interplay of thoughts, feelings, and behaviors."

Social awareness is also addressed in this program. It involves the ability to take the perspective of and empathize with others from diverse backgrounds and cultures in order to understand social and ethical norms of behavior and to recognize family, school, and community resources and supports. Skills like perspective-taking, empathy, respect for others, and demonstrating empathy and compassion, which are central to the interpersonal dimension of mentalization.

Relationship skills are also emphasized, including how to communicating effectively, how to developing positive relationships, how to practice teamwork and collaborative problem-solving, and resolving conflicts constructively, inherently relying on the ability to understand and respond to the mental states of others.

Responsible decision-making is another competency, which includes analyzing situations, identifying solutions for personal and social problems, and evaluating the benefits and consequences of various actions for personal, social, and collective well-being. This necessitates considering others' perspectives and potential emotional impacts on self and others.

The strengths of the CASEL framework provide a robust and widely adopted structure for SEL that implicitly supports many of the building blocks necessary for mentalization. Its explicit targeting of components, such as identifying one's own and others' feelings and fostering perspective-taking and empathy, lays a direct foundation for developing mentalizing skills. CASEL's emphasis on authentic school-family-community partnerships promotes the creation of broader supportive environments conducive to SEL development, which can indirectly support mentalization.

Despite these strengths, there are also limitations. The CASEL framework, widely recognized for its robust and comprehensive delineation of social and emotional competencies, has profoundly shaped the discourse and practice of SEL. Indeed, meta-analytic evidence consistently affirms the significant positive impact of school-based SEL interventions on student outcomes, from enhanced social–emotional skills and improved behavior to gains in academic performance (Durlak et al., 2011). However, the very ambition inherent in CASEL's broad framework, encompassing five core competencies, introduces complexities when translated into practical, deep implementation across diverse educational landscapes.

Historically, CASEL and generations of K-12 educational leaders have focused on individual student learning by prioritizing the development of discrete SEL skills within each student. This approach aimed to equip individual students with the internal tools to manage their emotions, understand themselves, build relationships, and make responsible decisions, thereby enhancing their personal academic and social adjustment. This individual-centric focus was promoted by the belief that a cumulative improvement in individual student capabilities would lead to enhanced academic outcomes, reduced behavioral issues, and greater personal well-being across the student population. It was also driven by practical considerations for classroom management and a desire to demonstrate measurable gains at the student level.

However, this singular focus faced several challenges. Primarily, it often overlooked the profound influence of systemic and environmental factors—such as overall school climate, the quality of teacher-student relationships, and broader societal contexts—on individual development. Consequently, the implementation of such programs could be inconsistent, heavily reliant on the training and commitment of individual educators and the availability of resources within specific schools. Furthermore, this emphasis on individual skill acquisition sometimes underestimated the dynamic and reciprocal interplay between individual and relational processes, which are fundamental to a holistic understanding of social–emotional development. This has led to an evolution in thinking toward more systemic SEL models that recognize the interwoven nature of individual capabilities and the supportive environments required to nurture them.

While the framework provides an invaluable guide, fully realizing its extensive scope in everyday classroom practice can be challenging. Reports on the current state of SEL implementation often highlight a tension between the framework's breadth and the depth of specific skill development achieved (Lawson et al., 2019). This can manifest as variations in pedagogical approaches, a focus on certain competencies over others, or a lack of explicit, consistent attention to more nuanced skills, such as truly differentiating between thoughts, feelings, and behaviors. Such disparities frequently stem from the demands of already crowded curricula, the need for sustained and high-quality professional development for educators, and varying levels of institutional commitment. Thus, while the efficacy of SEL is well-established, ensuring that the comprehensive vision of frameworks like CASEL translates into consistent, profound skill acquisition for all students remains a critical and ongoing area of focus in the field.

Promoting Alternative Thinking Strategies (PATHS)
Promoting Alternative Thinking Strategies

PATHS is a comprehensive universal prevention program designed for elementary school-aged children in grades K-6 (Greenberg & Kusche, 1993). Its primary aims are to promote emotional and social competencies, reduce aggression and behavior problems, and enhance the overall educational process within the classroom. The curriculum is structured around five core conceptual domains, which are integrated hierarchically: self-control, emotional understanding (often termed emotional literacy), positive self-esteem, relationships, and interpersonal problem-solving skills. A central tenet of the PATHS program is the principle that understanding and effectively regulating emotions are fundamental to successful problem-solving. The developers also assert that the program engages brain regions involved in social reasoning, emotions, and mentalizing.

Incorporation of mentalization principles in PATHS includes several elements that align with mentalization principles. The emotional understanding/literacy domain focuses on teaching children to identify, label, and understand a wide range of affective states. It emphasizes recognizing emotional cues in oneself and others, understanding the causes of emotions, and developing perspective-taking skills and specifically how and why to consider another person's point of view. This directly supports the mentalizing capacities of recognizing and understanding emotional states in both self and others.

Self-control lessons in this area teach children strategies to "stop and think" before acting, particularly when upset or facing conflict. This involves managing anger and frustration by linking emotional awareness to self-regulation techniques, which relates to the ability to manage one's own mental state to enable more thoughtful responses.

Interpersonal problem-solving is another component of this program that guides students through a structured process that includes identifying problems and associated feelings, setting goals, generating alternative solutions, anticipating the consequences of these solutions, and considering others' perspectives throughout the process. This requires students to mentalize the potential reactions, needs, and feelings of others involved in a given situation.

Strengths in developing mentalizing capacities in the PATHS curriculum explicitly aims to enhance children's ability to "recognize and interpret similarities and differences in the feelings, reactions and points of view of self and others." It provides systematic, developmentally-based lessons supported by materials such as "feeling faces cards" and scripted activities to reinforce emotional awareness and perspective-taking. The developers cite a substantial evidence base, with claims of over 40 published research studies documenting its effectiveness in improving emotional literacy, self-control, problem-solving skills, and reducing behavioral problems.

In terms of weaknesses, while the PATHS program makes a strong claim about engaging "mentalizing" brain networks, the explicit pedagogical focus within the curriculum materials appears to center more directly on emotional literacy, self-control techniques, and structured interpersonal problem-solving steps. The direct instruction on the more complex imaginative aspects of mentalization, such as inferring a wide range of intentional mental states (e.g., beliefs, desires, complex intentions beyond basic emotions or perspectives in a conflict), is less clearly articulated than the focus on emotions and overt problem-solving strategies.

Furthermore, research on the effectiveness of PATHS presents a mixed picture. While some sources and studies cited by the developers report significant positive impacts on various SEL outcomes and specific areas like reducing loneliness, reviews conducted by the What Works Clearinghouse (WWC), which apply rigorous standards for study inclusion, have found "no discernible effects" of PATHS on outcomes such as academic achievement, student social interactions, observed individual behavior, or student emotional status in the studies that met their criteria. This discrepancy is a critical consideration. "No discernible effects" in WWC terminology means that the qualifying evidence did not demonstrate statistically significant positive or negative effects, which does not definitively prove the program is ineffective in all aspects or contexts but rather that the evidence meeting their specific high standards did not show such effects (Institute of Education Sciences, n.d.).

Second Step Program

The Second Step program is a widely implemented, universal Tier 1 curriculum designed to teach "human skills" to students from early learning (preschool) through middle school (Moy & Hazen, 2018). Its core objectives include improving self-regulation, fostering social–emotional skills, such as emotion management, empathy, and kindness, and developing problem-solving abilities and executive functions. The program is structured with age-appropriate lessons and activities that evolve as students' progress through developmental stages.

In the early learning (PreK) program, the curriculum for preschoolers focuses on foundational skills, such as identifying and labeling basic emotions (e.g., happy, sad, surprised, scared, angry, worried, frustrated) in themselves and others. It introduces the concept that different people can have different feelings in the same situation, encourages caring and helping behaviors, and teaches strategies for naming feelings and managing common emotional challenges, like disappointment and anger. These concepts are often taught through engaging methods, like puppets, songs, and color photo weekly theme cards.

As students advance in elementary school, the program builds their emotion vocabulary and provides practice in identifying their own and others' emotions using behavioral cues (e.g., facial expressions, body language) and contextual information. Lessons explore how past experiences and unique perspectives can influence how individuals feel and respond to situations. A significant emphasis is placed on developing empathy through strategies for perspective-taking. Problem-solving components guide students to identify the wants and needs of others involved in a conflict. Instructional methods include role-play, discussions of authentic scenarios, personal reflection, and collaborative activities.

Strengths in the Second Step program offer direct instruction in identifying and labeling a range of emotions in oneself and others, which is a critical building block for mentalization. The program's explicit and consistent focus on empathy and perspective-taking directly addresses core components of interpersonal mentalization. Furthermore, the problem-solving units encourage students to consider the wants, needs, and viewpoints of others when navigating interpersonal conflicts, thereby promoting a mentalistic approach to social interactions. The curriculum is developmentally sequenced, ensuring that concepts are introduced in an age-appropriate manner from early learning through elementary and middle school. Some research indicates that Second Step can have positive effects on students' executive function skills and social skills and can lead to reductions in aggression.

The program's strength in fostering affective mentalization foundations is notable, as it heavily emphasizes recognizing, labeling, and understanding emotions, which are crucial for understanding the emotional worlds of self and others.

In terms of weaknesses, while Second Step effectively addresses many foundational skills related to mentalization, the term "mentalization" itself is not explicitly used in the program descriptions available. The curriculum clearly covers emotions and perspectives; however, the depth to which it guides students to explore more complex mental states—such as beliefs, intentions, desires, or phenomena like self-deception—or the intricate process of mentalizing (the imaginative, interpretive act of inferring these states) is not fully apparent from the provided materials. The program's framing of its content as "human skills" is accessible and likely resonates well with educators for broad adoption. This practical focus is a strength for implementation. However, this framing might inadvertently limit the exploration of the deeper, sometimes less conscious, and more complex internal processes that mentalization theory, particularly from a psychodynamic perspective, addresses (e.g., understanding unconscious motivations, preconscious biases in social interpretation). The program explicitly states it is "not psychotherapy," which is accurate and appropriate for a universal school-based curriculum. Yet a robust understanding of mentalization also draws from insights into the mind's complexities.

Research on the efficacy of Second Step has yielded varied results. While some studies show positive outcomes, particularly for earlier versions or specific populations, other research, including a study by Gottfredson et al. (2010) on an earlier edition, found no significant positive or negative effects on academic achievement or positive behaviors. Some analyses have indicated that many significant findings were moderated effects, meaning the program's impact varied depending on other factors. To deepen the mentalization aspect within the "human skills" framework, facilitators could be trained to guide discussions beyond surface-level skills. This would involve prompting students to explore the underlying thoughts, beliefs, and assumptions that drive emotions and behaviors in the scenarios presented, thereby touching on more complex mentalizing processes without needing to adopt a clinical framework.

The RULER Approach (Yale Center for Emotional Intelligence)

The RULER approach, developed at the Yale Center for Emotional Intelligence, is an evidence-based, systemic social and emotional learning (SEL) program designed for implementation from prekindergarten through 12th grade (Brackett et al., 2019). RULER is an acronym for the five core skills of emotional intelligence it aims to cultivate: recognizing emotions in oneself and others, understanding the causes and consequences of emotions, labeling emotions with a nuanced vocabulary, expressing emotions in accordance with cultural norms and social context, and regulating emotions with helpful strategies. The program utilizes four primary "Anchor Tools" that are embedded into the school's daily routines and practices:

The Charter is a collaboratively created document outlining how all members of the school community (students, teachers, staff) want to feel at school and the actions they will take to help each other experience those feelings. It fosters a positive emotional climate and shared behavioral expectations.

The Mood Meter is a visual tool that helps individuals identify, understand, and label their emotions based on two dimensions: energy (low to high) and pleasantness (unpleasant to pleasant). It expands emotional vocabulary and enhances self-awareness and the recognition of others' emotions.

The Meta-Moment is a step-by-step process that helps individuals pause, reflect, and make more thoughtful choices when they experience an emotional trigger, rather than reacting impulsively. It promotes emotional regulation and self-management.

The Blueprint is a tool designed for reflecting on conflicts and challenging interpersonal situations. It guides individuals to consider their own and others' perspectives, understand the emotional sequence of events, and develop strategies for resolving issues constructively, thereby supporting empathy and conflict resolution skills.

Systemic Emotional Intelligence and its Connection to Mentalization is part of the RULER's systemic approach that aims to infuse the principles of emotional intelligence into the very "immune system" of schools, influencing how students learn, teachers teach, families parent, and leaders lead. The RULER skills, particularly recognizing, understanding, and labeling emotions in oneself and others, are fundamental to mentalizing about affective states. The Mood Meter directly supports the identification and articulation of feelings, which is a prerequisite for reflecting on those feelings. The Blueprint, by prompting reflection on conflict and encouraging consideration of different perspectives, directly fosters aspects of interpersonal mentalization, such as understanding others' emotional experiences and potential motivations. The creation of an emotionally intelligent school climate through tools like the Charter provides a safe and common language, a crucial environmental factor for fostering mentalizing, as security is paramount for individuals to explore mental states.

Strengths in fostering emotional understanding and regulation as facets of mentalization provide a clear, memorable framework and a set of practical, versatile tools that facilitate the development of emotional literacy and regulation skills. Its systemic design, involving all school stakeholders—staff, students, and families—promotes a consistent emotional climate and shared understanding across the school community. Research has shown that RULER can lead to positive shifts in school climate, improved teacher instruction and classroom organization, increased student engagement and academic performance (particularly in English language arts), better work habits, reduced rates of bullying and aggressive behavior, and enhanced social skills and leadership qualities among students. These outcomes are highly conducive to, and often rely upon, developing mentalizing capacities.

While there is significant overlap between EI and mentalization, particularly concerning the understanding and regulation of emotions, mentalization theory as articulated by Fonagy and colleagues also places strong emphasis on understanding a broader range of intentional mental states (such as beliefs, desires, intentions, and goals) and the developmental, often preconscious, aspects of how individuals interpret themselves and others. The RULER curriculum, while excellent for emotional literacy, may not explicitly delve into these more complex cognitive and developmental dimensions of mentalization with the same depth as its focus on emotions. This could be considered one of its weaknesses. For instance, while the RULER skills are vital, mentalization also involves the imaginative inference of others' beliefs and intentions, which might be distinct from or even contradictory to their expressed emotions. It also involves understanding how one's own mind, with its inherent biases and past experiences, shapes these interpretations. The RULER tools, while powerful for emotional understanding, may not inherently prompt students to this deeper level of inferential reasoning about nonemotional mental states or the complexities of intersubjectivity without explicit pedagogical guidance. The ongoing efficacy trial for high school RULER aims to assess its impact on emotion skills, school climate, engagement, and well-being, which are related to mentalization but are not direct measures of mentalizing capacity itself.

To leverage RULER for more comprehensive mentalization development, educators could be trained to use the RULER tools as springboards for discussions that extend beyond emotions to explore underlying beliefs, intentions, and perspectives.

Facing History and Ourselves (FHAO)

Since 1976, Facing History and Ourselves (FHAO) has distinguished itself as a highly regarded educational organization, leveraging the study of historical events—particularly those involving genocide and human rights violations—to cultivate civic engagement, empathy, and ethical reasoning in middle and high school students. In contrast to many more generalized SEL programs, FHAO's curriculum adopts a deeply psychologically-minded approach. It actively prompts students to grapple with moral dilemmas and consider their own societal roles through dynamic, interactive methods, including robust discussions and critical analysis of primary sources. The organization also provides extensive professional development for educators, consistently reporting high satisfaction rates among participants. Research has indicated that engagement with FHAO programs leads to significant improvements in students' historical understanding, tolerance, civic efficacy, prosocial behavior, and overall school climate. While the sensitive nature of the subject matter necessitates skilled facilitation and access to resources can sometimes present a challenge for certain schools, FHAO is widely viewed as a transformative initiative, expertly weaving historical analysis with social–emotional learning to equip students to confront injustice in their own communities and the wider world (Perron, 2014).

Anna Freud National Centre for Children and Families (AFNCCF) Programs

The Anna Freud National Centre for Children and Families (AFNCCF) is a leading institution in the development, research, and dissemination of mentalization-based treatment (MBT) and mentalization-informed approaches for children, young people, and families. Their work is explicitly grounded in the theory of mentalization as elaborated by Peter Fonagy and his colleagues.

Mentalization-based treatment for children (MBT-C) is a time-limited, transdiagnostic therapy designed for children aged 5–12 experiencing emotional and behavioral difficulties, anxiety, or depression. It involves weekly individual child sessions integrated with parent sessions, aiming to build mentalizing abilities by focusing on foundational elements like attention control, emotion regulation, and explicit mentalizing.

Mentalization-based treatment for adolescents (MBT-A) is tailored for adolescents presenting with interpersonal difficulties, emotional dysregulation, impulsivity, and self-harm. It aims to enhance their capacity to accurately represent their own and others' feelings, especially in emotionally challenging situations.

Introductory mentalization courses provides self-guided online training courses that offer a foundational understanding of mentalization theory and its applications for professionals working with children, young people, and families. These courses often serve as prerequisites for more specialized MBT training.

School-based interventions and research: the Centre is actively involved in research on mental health in schools. A notable example is the "Education for Wellbeing" trial, conducted in partnership with UCL, which evaluated several school-based interventions. This trial found the "Strategies for Safety and Wellbeing" (SSW) intervention to be particularly promising. SSW is a mental health awareness approach that helps students normalize everyday emotions (like stress and sadness), better understand how to differentiate them from mental ill health, and know where to access support if needed.

Training for schools and colleges: AFNCCF offers a variety of training courses for education staff on topics such as responding to self-harm, senior mental health leadership, school attendance and mental well-being, peer support, digital resilience, autism, antiracism and mental health, staff well-being, and reflective practice and supervision.

Direct Application of Mentalization Theory and Promotion of Reflective Capacity

A core strength of AFNCCF programs is their direct and explicit grounding in mentalization theory. The "mentalizing stance"—characterized by curiosity, a "not-knowing" approach, empathy, and validation—is central to all MBT approaches and is a key skill taught to practitioners. These interventions aim to help individuals make sense of themselves and others in terms of underlying mental states (thoughts, feelings, intentions). Furthermore, specific training programs, such as "reflective practice and supervision training" for school staff, directly target the development of reflective capacity, which is integral to mentalizing. This focus on the educator's or therapist's own mentalizing stance as crucial for facilitating mentalization in others is a distinguishing feature. Additionally, these approaches aim to build "epistemic trust"—the trust in the authenticity and personal relevance of interpersonally transmitted knowledge—which (Fonagy and Allison, 2014) argue is vital for learning and therapeutic change.

Strengths: Deep Theoretical Grounding and Focus on Reflective Practice

The most significant strength of AFNCCF's offerings in this context is their profound and direct theoretical link to the concept of mentalization. The emphasis on the practitioner's (and by extension, the educator's) own mentalizing stance as a critical component of effective intervention is paramount. The SSW intervention, emerging from their research, demonstrates evidence of improving mental health literacy and, for some student groups, reducing emotional difficulties, offering a pragmatic way to introduce mentalizing principles universally.

While deeply rooted in robust theory, adapting these approaches for universal implementation in general educational settings presents challenges. MBT itself is primarily a therapeutic model, often intensive and requiring specialized, ongoing training and supervision for practitioners to achieve competency. Translating its nuanced principles for use by general educators in a classroom setting requires careful consideration to maintain the core tenets while ensuring feasibility and appropriateness. Short training courses alone are unlikely to equip educators with sufficient skills; sustained support and supervision are key, which has significant resource implications for schools. Historically, research into psychoanalytic and mentalization-based approaches in schools has also faced obstacles related to funding, ethical complexities, participant recruitment, and sometimes practitioner resistance to empirical research methodologies.

However, the "mentalizing stance" itself—being curious about a student's internal world, adopting a "not-knowing" position rather than making assumptions, and validating their experiences—is a highly transferable principle. Training educators in this stance could be a powerful, universally applicable strategy to create mentalization-fostering classrooms, even without implementing a full MBT curriculum. This approach shifts the focus from mere behavior management to understanding the mind behind the behavior. Furthermore, interventions like SSW, which focus on normalizing emotions and promoting help-seeking, serve as a pragmatic bridge between complex clinical mentalization models and universal prevention in schools. SSW and similar psychoeducational approaches grounded in mentalizing principles (i.e., understanding and normalizing inner experiences) offer a scalable way to introduce foundational mentalizing concepts into the broader school population, potentially serving as a Tier 1 intervention that complements more intensive supports for students who require them. This helps address the challenge of adapting sophisticated clinical models for widespread educational use.

The Anna Freud National Centre for Children and Families (AFNCCF), particularly Peter Fonagy's efforts to embed mentalization in K-12 education, offers a pivotal expansion for this paper's core argument. Recent empirical findings from this European research group move beyond theoretical constructs, powerfully illustrating the practical benefits of mentalizing capacities within educational settings. A series of recent studies by Schwarzer et al. (2023, 2024a, 2024b) lend robust empirical weight to mentalization's role in well-being for educators and young adults alike. For instance, Schwarzer et al. (2024a) discovered that both mentalizing capacity and self-efficacy significantly predict well-being and can lessen symptom severity among novice special education teachers, suggesting mentalization might actually serve as a protective shield against occupational stress. Building on this, a longitudinal study by Schwarzer et al. (2024b) found that higher mentalizing abilities in young adults foreshadow improved well-being and more adaptive ways of regulating emotions over time, underscoring its foundational link to individual emotional health. Furthermore, Schwarzer et al. (2023) showed that mentalizing partially mediates the connection between attachment insecurity and overall stress levels in preservice teachers, highlighting its potential to buffer the negative effects of insecure attachment and cultivate greater resilience in future educators. Taken together, these studies affirm that mentalization isn't just an abstract concept; it's a measurable skill with tangible, positive consequences for individual resilience, emotional regulation, and overall flourishing. The AFNCCF's intentional focus on integrating mentalization into school systems, evident in Fonagy's current collaborations, represents a critical stride forward. This work signals a profound shift: it recognizes mentalizing as fundamental to both academic achievement and holistic development, rather than treating mental health as separate from educational outcomes. Including these findings significantly strengthens the argument that a mentalization-informed approach provides a more robust and clinically grounded path to fostering effective citizenry, directly addressing the essential capacities needed for navigating complex social realities, managing one's own internal states, and engaging empathetically with others.

The Civic Opportunity Gap: Trauma, Poverty, and the Capacity to Mentalize

While the educational frameworks discussed earlier offer promising pathways for civic renewal, we must confront a stark reality: the opportunity to develop mentalizing capacity is not distributed equally. There is a "civic opportunity gap" that mirrors the economic and academic achievement gaps in our society. This gap is fundamentally rooted in the neurobiology of stress and trauma.

Mentalization is a phylogenetically recent and fragile capacity. It resides largely in the prefrontal cortex, the part of the brain most sensitive to stress. When an individual is in a state of high arousal—triggered by fear, hunger, violence, or chronic instability—the brain switches control from the reflective prefrontal cortex to the reactive amygdala. In this "fight-or-flight" mode, mentalization shuts down. This is an adaptive survival mechanism; if one is being chased by a predator, one needs to run, not reflect on the predator's childhood.

However, for students living in conditions of chronic poverty, systemic racism, or community violence, this "threat state" can become a baseline setting. A child who does not know where their next meal is coming from, or who navigates a neighborhood where safety is not guaranteed, is forced to remain in a state of hypervigilance. Their cognitive resources are dedicated to scanning for threats, leaving little surplus energy for the "luxury" of contemplating the mental states of others or engaging in abstract civic reflection.

Therefore, implementing mentalization-focused civics education requires a trauma-informed approach. We cannot demand that students "mentalize" if we have not first established a sense of safety. This means that social policy—including nutrition support, safe housing, and the dismantling of systemic discrimination—is, in fact, civic policy. We cannot build a reflective citizenry on a foundation of chronic toxic stress. Educational programs must be coupled with "wrap-around" services that lower the physiological stress levels of students. Only when the body is safe can the mind afford to be curious. Addressing the material conditions of students' lives is not separate from their civic education; it is the physiological prerequisite for it.

Supporting Evidence

A growing body of research, spanning diverse age groups and innovative modalities, confirms that these critical social–cognitive skills are amenable to deliberate instruction and practice. Interventions in early childhood education have shown particular promise. For instance, the SAGA Project in Finland developed and implemented a mentalization-based program for preschool settings, leveraging shared storybook reading combined with mentalizing dialogues. This approach not only facilitated significant gains in young children's social–emotional development but also enhanced the mentalizing skills of their teachers, highlighting a dual benefit (Marttunen et al., 2020).

Similarly, an innovative European program designed to bolster children's social and emotional learning in preschools yielded notable improvements in both theory of mind (ToM) and emotion understanding among participants, underscoring the potential of structured interventions at foundational developmental stages (Lecce et al., 2014). This instructional capacity extends into primary education, as evidenced by a training program for 7–8-year-olds that effectively enhanced their advanced ToM abilities, demonstrating that these complex social–cognitive skills can be actively refined beyond early childhood (Lecce et al., 2017).

Even in challenging contexts, such as among low-income preschoolers in the United States, targeted storybook interactions focusing on characters' mental states led to measurable improvements in ToM understanding, indicating the adaptability and accessibility of such methods across socioeconomic strata (Miskowiec & Bloom, 2016). The cumulative impact of these efforts is further corroborated by broader analyses. A comprehensive meta-analysis of various ToM training programs, encompassing numerous controlled studies, conclusively found that these interventions consistently led to substantial improvements in children's ToM skills when compared to control groups, providing robust empirical support for their overall efficacy (Grosse et al., 2017). Beyond traditional pedagogical methods, technological advancements are also proving instrumental. A pilot study exploring a virtual reality (VR) application designed to teach ToM skills to children aged 5–6 years demonstrated promising results, suggesting that immersive digital environments could offer novel and engaging pathways for mentalizing skill development (Parsons et al., 2017).

Collectively, these investigations provide compelling empirical grounding for the deliberate integration of mentalization-focused activities into educational curricula. They underscore that mentalizing is not merely an innate capacity but a cultivable skill, essential for fostering children's social and emotional development and, by extension, their capacity for engaged and ethical citizenry. The cultivation of these capacities from early childhood through adolescence is fundamental for nurturing individuals who can participate meaningfully in a democratic society, characterized by empathy, understanding, and constructive dialogue.

Chapter 8

Engaging Parents and the Wider Community

For educators, their own ability to mentalize—to understand their own mental states and those of their students—is pivotal in creating effective, responsive, and supportive learning environments that can cater to diverse student needs. When teachers can accurately interpret the underlying reasons for a student's behavior (e.g., understanding that disengagement might stem from anxiety or confusion rather than defiance), they can respond more empathetically and constructively.

Enhanced mentalizing skills in students contribute directly to their ability to manage their emotions more effectively and to resolve interpersonal conflicts in a more constructive manner. This, in turn, helps to foster classroom climates that are more secure, empathetic, and conducive to learning. Students who feel understood by their teachers and peers are more likely to engage positively in the learning process. Furthermore, mentalization is essential for building and maintaining healthy interpersonal relationships, improving communication, and enhancing psychosocial well-being in general. Conversely, a lack of mentalizing ability can lead to difficulties in social adaptation, challenges in overcoming stress, and an increased vulnerability to various adjustment problems.

Fostering a Mentalizing School Ethos: Educator Training and Whole-School Initiatives

For mentalization to truly take root in educational settings, it cannot be confined to isolated lessons; it must permeate the entire school ethos. This requires a commitment to educator training and whole-school initiatives.

Educator training: teachers and other school staff are pivotal in creating mentalization-fostering environments. Training should equip them with a solid understanding of the core principles of mentalization and the practical application of a "mentalizing stance"—an attitude of curiosity, empathy, and a willingness to explore the student's internal world without premature judgment or assumption. Awareness of their own attachment patterns and mentalizing tendencies, and how these can influence their interactions in the classroom and their responses to students, particularly those exhibiting challenging behaviors, is also an important characteristic for teachers to possess.

DOI: 10.4324/9781003771296-8

Practical strategies for responding to challenging behaviors from a mentalizing perspective, which involves looking beyond the behavior to understand the underlying thoughts, feelings, and needs of the student, is also very important. The teacher, in many respects, serves as the primary "mentalizing other" for students within the school context. Mentalization develops in relationships where a more mature mind reflects on and helps to make sense of a child's internal state. If educators are not themselves mentalizing effectively or lack the training to foster it, student-focused curricula will likely have limited impact. Therefore, investing in robust, ongoing professional development that supports educators' own mentalizing capacity is not merely about curriculum delivery but about transforming their way of relating to and understanding students.

Whole-school initiatives that embed mentalizing language and concepts are also crucially important. The principles of mentalization should be woven into the school's culture, mission, and daily practices. This can involve adopting a shared language around feelings, thoughts, and perspectives. Promoting reflective practice structures that support staff reflection, such as peer supervision groups or dedicated time for reflective dialogue about student interactions and classroom dynamics, are also crucially important. This helps educators process their experiences, refine their mentalizing skills, and support each other.

Creating safe and secure environments is another fundamental prerequisite for mentalizing because it provides a sense of safety and security. Schools must prioritize creating environments where students feel physically and emotionally safe, respected, and comfortable exploring and expressing their thoughts and feelings without fear of punitive or dismissive responses.

The Role of Secure Relationships and a "Not-Knowing Stance" in the Classroom

The quality of relationships within the classroom is paramount for fostering mentalization. Secure teacher-student relationships, characterized by trust, consistency, and emotional availability, provide the relational safety net that supports students' capacity to mentalize. Building on this, educators are encouraged to adopt a "not-knowing stance." This involves approaching students with genuine curiosity about their internal worlds, rather than making quick assumptions or imposing adult interpretations. It means asking open-ended questions, listening attentively, and working collaboratively with the student to understand their experience.

This "not-knowing stance" presents a pedagogical paradox: the educator, often seen as the expert, deliberately adopts a position of uncertainty to foster deeper knowing in the student (Proctor et al., 2021). This approach can create a space where students feel safe to explore their own minds and are invited to become active collaborators in making sense of their experiences. It avoids the pitfall of the adult imposing an interpretation, which can lead to superficial compliance or a "pseudo-mentalizing," where the student parrots what they think the adult wants to hear, rather than engaging in genuine self-reflection. Educators may require support and training to become comfortable with this level of uncertainty and to recognize it not as a lack of competence but as a powerful tool for fostering authentic self-understanding and robust mentalizing skills in their students. Crucially, even when a student's behavior is problematic, validating their underlying emotional experience can be a vital first step before exploring alternative behaviors.

The development of mentalization is profoundly relational and extends beyond the school walls. To create a truly mentalizing environment around a child, efforts within the school must be complemented by engagement with parents and the wider community. Providing resources, workshops, and information for parents on the principles of mentalization and reflective parenting can help them support their child's development of these skills at home. When schools, families, and community organizations work in partnership, they create more consistent and mutually reinforcing environments that support children's social and emotional learning. If mentalizing is only fostered at school but not understood or reinforced in other key areas of a child's life, its impact may be diluted.

CARE: An Educator's SEL Program

A particularly relevant program to consider in the context of fostering educator well-being and their capacities for attunement is CARE, an educator SEL program developed by Mark Greenberg and Tish Jennings, who also codeveloped the well-known PATHS program (Greenberg & Jennings, n.d.). This initiative directly addresses the critical need to support the social–emotional competence of the adults within the school system, a point I've aptly identified as fundamentally important. CARE aligns significantly with the proposals for cultivating educators' mentalizing capacities and overall well-being. Its focus on enhancing teachers' own social–emotional skills and resilience directly resonates with the argument that educators require robust emotional regulation and self-awareness to effectively model and nurture these qualities in students. By integrating practices like mindfulness, CARE inherently supports the development of self-awareness and the ability to recognize one's own internal states—foundational elements of mentalization. When educators are more present and regulated, they are better equipped to perceive and respond sensitively to students' emotional and mental states, a cornerstone of a truly mentalizing classroom environment. Ultimately, the program posits that supporting the internal world of the educator indirectly yet powerfully benefits students by fostering more supportive and effective learning climates.

In a somewhat different light, my major premise posits that democracy faces a significant crisis, marked by an erosion of the collective capacity for discerning truth and engaging in constructive civic discourse. I argue that the cultivation of mentalization is integral to revitalizing genuine community participation, as healthy civic life profoundly depends on quality interaction underpinned by these crucial skills—encompassing empathy, perspective-taking, effective communication, and conflict regulation, all of which contribute to building essential social capital and trust. Seen through this lens, CARE shares significant common ground with what I am suggesting, even as its immediate focus differs. The kinship between CARE and my proposal lies fundamentally in the shared recognition that systemic health—be it a classroom environment or a functioning democracy—is largely predicated upon the robust inner capacities of its individual members. CARE, by intentionally nurturing educators' social–emotional competence, self-awareness, and resilience, strengthens the very human infrastructure of schools. Just as this paper argues that a citizenry capable of mentalizing is essential for productive democratic discourse, CARE acts on the principle that mentally attuned and regulated teachers are crucial for creating a learning environment conducive to healthy interaction and student development. It addresses the well-being of the "enablers" of learning, implicitly acknowledging that a reflective, emotionally regulated adult is better equipped to foster the very capacities we seek to cultivate in students for future civic life. The program's emphasis on mindfulness, for example, directly enhances the self-awareness vital for mentalization, which then extends to improved attunement with others in the classroom. That said, the primary divergence resides in the explicit target and theoretical framing of the intervention. While CARE offers profound benefits to the educator's internal world, operating primarily within the broader SEL and mindfulness frameworks, my central argument is a more direct call for the cultivation of mentalization as a core capacity among citizens themselves to address a societal crisis of democratic participation. My proposal advocates for a broader societal application of mentalization to foster "quality interaction" in civic spaces, whereas CARE's specific focus is on enabling educators to create optimal learning environments. Ultimately, however, a program like CARE is not a departure from my suggestion but rather a compelling and empirically supported example of a necessary component. It underscores the profound importance of tending to the mentalizing capacities of key societal actors—in this case, educators—as a foundational step toward fostering the reflective, empathetic citizenry essential for a vibrant democracy.

The Evolution of School Climate: From Individual Skills to Systemic Ecology

A truly mentalizing school ethos stands as a critical understanding for educational effectiveness, reflecting a profound shift in the field's thinking regarding social and emotional learning. Early proponents of social and emotional learning (SEL) in the late 1990s often concentrated on teaching discrete SEL skills within individual classrooms. Over time, however, a deeper realization gained traction: that effective learning hinges not just on acquiring individual skills but also on developing new understandings and, crucially, on the synergistic power of a supportive, school-wide culture. This evolution led to what is now often termed "SEL 2.0" or "systemic SEL," a deliberate pairing of individual and relational experiences with the broader social norms, expectations, and values that define a school's environment.

This systemic view, frequently referred to as school climate, reflects an ecologically informed understanding, much like Urie Bronfenbrenner's model, which recognizes that human development is profoundly shaped by nested systems—from individual interactions to larger group dynamics within a school. This progression toward a systemic perspective finds robust support in seminal work within school climate research. Cohen et al. (2009) offered a comprehensive overview, defining school climate not merely as atmosphere but as the intricate quality and character of school life itself. They highlighted its multifaceted nature, encompassing norms, goals, values, interpersonal relationships, and teaching practices, asserting that a positive climate forms the bedrock for academic success, healthy development, and civic engagement.

Building upon this foundation, Thapa et al. (2013) reviewed the extensive body of school climate research, reinforcing its conceptualization as a complex construct. Their synthesis underscored the strong empirical links between a positive school climate and improved student outcomes—ranging from enhanced learning and well-being to reduced behavioral challenges. Both reviews affirm that a healthy school climate functions as an active, pervasive force, influencing every member of the school community. Such a systemic understanding profoundly informs the concept of a "mentalizing school ethos." A school truly committed to mentalization cannot merely teach perspective-taking in isolated lessons; instead, it must embed relational safety, mutual respect, and a genuine curiosity about others' internal states into its very fabric.

This means that mentalizing principles should permeate administrative policies, shape teacher-student interactions, guide peer dynamics, and even influence the physical environment, collectively creating a consistent "container" for emotional and cognitive reflection. When a school operates with such a pervasive mentalizing ethos, it amplifies the impact of individual skill-building, cultivating a powerfully supportive environment where the development of mentalizing capacities is not just taught but consistently lived and reinforced. The fundamental importance of secure relationships and adopting a "not-knowing stance" in the classroom further underscores this systemic approach. These elements are, indeed, vital components of a mentalizing environment, fostering the psychological safety necessary for genuine inquiry and understanding among all members of the school community.

Short-Term Scaffolding: Building Mentalization in the Public Square

Beyond the generational project of transforming K-12 education, the urgent state of our democratic crisis demands short-term interventions that can scaffold mentalizing capacities and rebuild epistemic trust among the current adult citizenry. While the comprehensive educational framework proposed in this book acts as the long-term preventative medicine, we must also identify and support immediate "prosthetic" environments—settings that artificially induce or support mentalization when the natural capacity has been degraded by polarization. These short-term solutions do not require a return to school but rather the infusion of mentalizing principles into the institutions where adults currently spend their lives: workplaces, community centers, and local governance bodies.

One immediate avenue for restoring epistemic trust lies in the structured application of deliberative democracy initiatives, such as citizens' assemblies. Unlike traditional town halls, which often devolve into shouting matches that reinforce splitting and projection, deliberative forums are designed with specific rules of engagement that mirror the conditions necessary for mentalization. In these settings, moderators act as the "mentalizing other," ensuring that participants explain the values behind their positions rather than merely attacking opponents. This structure forces a pause in reactive thinking, allowing for "hot mentalization" to occur in a safe container. By participating in these controlled environments, citizens can experience a temporary restoration of trust—a "lived experience" that disagreement does not equal existential threat. This creates a feedback loop where the safety of the process allows for the lowering of epistemic hypervigilance, enabling the intake of new information.

Furthermore, the corporate and organizational sector offers a vital, underutilized arena for short-term mentalization training. The concept of "psychological safety," widely popularized in modern management theory, is functionally synonymous with a mentalizing environment. Short-term interventions in workplaces that focus on conflict resolution, "perspective-taking" leadership, and emotional regulation are not merely productivity tools; they are civic exercises. When an organization trains its employees to interpret a colleague's failure not as malice (a non-mentalizing stance) but as a result of context or stress, they are exercising the same muscle required to interpret a political opponent's motives. Expanding these programs to explicitly label these skills as civic assets could provide a rapid, scalable way to reintroduce mentalization to the adult population.

Contextualizing the Framework Within Broader Civic Efforts

Contextualizing the proposed K-12 framework within these broader efforts is essential for understanding its true scope. The educational reform proposed in this book should not be viewed as a solitary silo but rather as the foundational layer of a multitiered civic infrastructure. It aligns with and reinforces existing movements toward restorative justice, which replaces punitive, behaviorist approaches to crime with processes that demand the mentalization of the victim and the offender. In a restorative justice circle, the offender must confront the internal reality of the victim, a profound exercise in empathy and theory of mind that serves the community far better than retribution.

This framework also complements the growing field of "constructive journalism," which seeks to report news not through conflict-framing (which triggers tribalism) but through complexity-framing. Traditional sensation-based journalism often encourages a "teleological" mode of thinking, where actions are judged only by their visible outcomes. Constructive journalism, by helping readers understand the why behind societal events and the internal motivations of different actors, acts as a form of mass-media mentalization.

By viewing the K-12 initiative as the foundation and these community, corporate, and media interventions as the superstructure, we establish a comprehensive ecosystem for democratic renewal. The school system generates a future citizenry with a robust, innate capacity for mentalization, while deliberative forums, restorative practices, and psychologically aware workplaces provide the necessary scaffolding to hold the fractured psyche of the current polity together. In this way, the project of rebuilding epistemic trust becomes a shared societal endeavor, bridging the gap between the classroom and the public square.

Chapter 9

Key Insights From Program Analyses

The analysis of prominent educational programs reveals a varied landscape regarding the integration of mentalization. While many social and emotional learning (SEL) programs, such as those aligned with the CASEL framework, PATHS, Second Step, and RULER, effectively address essential components related to mentalization—notably emotional literacy, empathy, and perspective-taking—the explicitness, depth, and direct theoretical grounding in mentalization per se differ considerably. These programs provide strong foundational skills.

Initiatives stemming from the Anna Freud National Centre for Children and Families, with their explicit basis in mentalization-based treatment principles, offer pathways for deeper and more direct mentalization work, particularly through the cultivation of a mentalizing stance in educators and targeted interventions like Strategies for Safety and Wellbeing (SSW). However, the challenge often lies in adapting clinically derived models for universal application in diverse educational contexts without diluting their core efficacy (Bak, 2015).

Addressing Research Gaps Longitudinal Impact Studies

There is a pressing need for more longitudinal research that tracks the long-term effects of integrated critical thinking, SEL, and mentalization-informed civic education programs. Such studies should follow students from K-12 through higher education and into adulthood to assess impacts on their civic engagement patterns, political participation levels, democratic dispositions, and overall contributions to community life. While some longitudinal evidence suggests positive outcomes, more robust and extended studies are required to validate and refine current approaches.

Intersectionality and Equity

Future research must more deeply investigate how different pedagogical approaches to critical thinking and mentalization differentially impact students from diverse socioeconomic, racial, ethnic, linguistic, and cultural backgrounds. A key focus should be on identifying and evaluating strategies that effectively address and mitigate the "civic opportunity gap," ensuring that all students, particularly those from

DOI: 10.4324/9781003771296-9

historically marginalized communities, have access to high-quality civic learning experiences that empower them for full democratic participation. This includes critical research on program implementation and outcomes in diverse settings.

Role of Digital Technologies

The rapidly evolving landscape of digital technologies and social media platforms necessitates ongoing research into their impact on youth civic development. This includes further exploration of the efficacy of interventions designed to foster critical digital literacy, resilience to online misinformation and manipulation, and the capacity for empathic and constructive engagement in online civic spaces. Understanding how to leverage technology for positive civic learning while mitigating its risks is a critical research frontier.

Teacher Development and Support

More research is needed to identify and validate effective models of preservice and in-service professional development that genuinely equip educators with the confidence, competence, and ongoing support required to implement these complex pedagogical strategies. This is particularly important for teachers working in challenging or politically polarized environments, who may face unique pressures and require specialized skills in facilitating difficult conversations and managing classroom dynamics.

Psychoanalytic Contributions

Further empirical and theoretical work is encouraged to explore how psychoanalytic concepts can be practically applied, adapted, and validated within educational settings to enhance students' and educators' mentalization capacities related to civic issues, intergroup relations, and unconscious group dynamics. While conceptually rich, more research is needed on the tangible impact and practical implementation of these ideas in K-12 civics education to move beyond theoretical articulation toward evidence-based practice.

Conclusion

A Review of Prominent Educational Programs and Psychoanalytic Schools that Could Bolster Civic Engagement

The recommendations put forth in this paper advocate for a systemic and holistic approach to civic development. Enhancing critical thinking requires embedding complex societal issues in the curriculum, promoting deliberative pedagogies, integrating media and digital literacy, and facilitating action civics projects. Crucially, educators need sustained professional development to effectively teach these skills and navigate the complexities of political polarization in the classroom. Assessment practices must also evolve to measure higher-order thinking skills beyond rote memorization. Similarly, cultivating mentalization and social–emotional competencies necessitates the explicit integration of SEL frameworks in civic contexts, with a clear connection between SEL skills and democratic practices. Pedagogies that foster empathy, perspective-taking, and the ability to engage in constructive dialogue across differences are essential. Creating supportive school environments that prioritize well-being and leverage positive peer interactions can further contribute to the development of prosocial self-identities crucial for engaged citizenship. Achieving these goals requires robust systemic and institutional supports. K-12 schools must become hubs for democratic practice, fostering student agency and participation. Universities, media organizations, law enforcement, and psychoanalytic institutes all have vital collaborative roles to play in supporting holistic civic development. Policy recommendations must prioritize and fund comprehensive civic education, address the civic opportunity gap, and support ongoing research and evaluation. Looking ahead, future research should focus on longitudinal impact studies, the intersectionality of these competencies and equity, the role of digital technologies, teacher development and support, and the practical application of psychoanalytic insights in educational settings. Fostering communities of practice across sectors and committing to iterative improvement are essential for advancing this agenda. The cultivation of critical and mentally astute democratic citizens is not merely an educational goal but a fundamental necessity for the survival and flourishing of democratic societies. By recognizing the distinct yet interconnected power of mentalization and critical thinking, and by implementing the comprehensive recommendations outlined in this paper, we can empower individuals to engage with the complexities of the world with understanding, reason, and a deep commitment to democratic values. This integrated approach holds the

DOI: 10.4324/9781003771296-10

transformative potential to strengthen our civic fabric, foster more inclusive and productive dialogue, and ultimately contribute to a more just and resilient democracy for all.

On a more psychoanalytic and community-based level, there are also organizations like the Alliance for Psychoanalytic Schools (APS) that support institutions applying these principles. These schools operate on the belief that a deep understanding of the child's inner world, emotions, and relationships is fundamental to their intellectual and social development (Streeter, n.d.).

The Alliance for Psychoanalytic Schools (APS) is a nonprofit organization that provides support and a forum for a small network of educational institutions that integrate psychoanalytic and developmental principles into their mission. These schools are characterized by a deep respect for the child's inner world, a focus on the emotional aspects of learning, and the use of behavior as a form of communication. They are not merely traditional schools with therapists on staff; their entire pedagogical approach is informed by psychoanalytic concepts, such as the importance of the parent-child relationship and the significance of emotional states in development.

Psychoanalytic schools, however, are far from common. The APS includes a small number of member schools, and while their influence is notable, they represent a very niche and specialized approach to education. Creating a new psychoanalytic school is a complex and resource-intensive undertaking. It would require more than just a curriculum; it would necessitate a fundamental shift in institutional culture. The staff, from teachers to administrators, would need extensive training to understand and apply psychoanalytic principles. This training would likely be intensive and long-term, focusing on their own capacity for mentalization and emotional attunement. The financial model would also need to be sustainable, as this approach often involves a lower student-to-teacher ratio and a greater emphasis on individual and family support.

This development, if it were to become more widespread, would be profoundly important for reimagining our democracy. A society's civic health is not just about its laws and institutions but about the psychological capacities of its citizens. This type of educational model would directly cultivate the skills that are essential for a healthy democracy: empathy, perspective-taking, emotional regulation, and a tolerance for ambiguity. By teaching children to mentalize and to understand the "whys" behind behavior from a young age, these schools would be preparing a new generation to engage in constructive dialogue, to see opponents not as enemies but as complex individuals, and to build the kind of genuine community that this book outlines.

Bridging the Gap: Immediate Practices for a Mentalizing Society

While the systemic educational reforms advocated in this book represent a long-term generational project, we must also address the immediate needs of the current moment. We cannot wait twenty years for a new generation to save us; we must begin to build the necessary psychological musculature today. To that end, the principles of mentalization and epistemic trust can be translated into manageable, daily habits for parents, educators, and concerned citizens—short-term interventions that function as "cognitive speed bumps" in our fast-paced, reactive culture.

To bolster mentalization, for example, educators and parents can adopt simple, consistent reflective prompts. When discussing a news event or a social conflict, we can pause to ask questions such as "What might the person on the other side of this issue be feeling or thinking?" or "What life experiences might lead someone to hold that strong opinion?" These questions do not require us to agree with the opposing view. Instead, they encourage the practice of seeing others as having valid, separate minds with their own internal logic. This simple act of perspective-taking, even when brief, interrupts the cycle of reactive certainty and begins to build the cognitive empathy at the heart of mentalization.

Similarly, epistemic trust can be cultivated through daily habits of critical consumption. A short-term classroom exercise or a dinner table discussion might involve a "two-source check" for any provocative online claim or a game of "spotting the emotion"—identifying whether a piece of content is designed to inform us or to provoke a specific emotional reaction like outrage or fear. These small interventions are not a panacea, but they slow down the automatic acceptance or rejection of information. They foster a more deliberate, trusting, and verifiable relationship with knowledge sources, allowing us to navigate the information landscape with agency rather than anxiety.

The "Good Enough" Citizen: A Winnicottian Goal for Democracy

As we envision the outcomes of this educational framework, we must guard against the allure of perfectionism. The goal of a mentalizing democracy is not to produce a utopia of perfectly rational, endlessly empathetic citizens who never succumb to tribalism or anger. Such a goal is inconsistent with human nature. Instead, we might borrow again from D.W. Winnicott, who coined the term "the good-enough mother." Winnicott argued that a child does not need a perfect parent; they need a parent who is reliable, generally attuned, and capable of repairing ruptures when they inevitably occur.

Similarly, a healthy democracy requires "good-enough citizens." A good-enough citizen is not one who never feels the pull of prejudice or the comfort of the echo chamber. Rather, they are one who possesses the psychological capacity to recognize when they have regressed. They are capable of "repair"—of returning to a mentalizing stance after a moment of failure. The K-12 curriculum proposed here aims to instill this capacity for repair. We are building a citizenry that can survive the inevitable conflicts of a pluralistic society not by avoiding them but by having the resilience to work through them without losing sight of the humanity of the other.

Zooming Out: The Ripple Effect of the Mentalizing Citizen

Ultimately, these immediate techniques and the broader K-12 curriculum are not separate endeavors; they are part of a unified movement toward civic maturity. When we zoom out and imagine a generation of students who have been immersed in this program, the potential impact on our wider democratic institutions becomes staggering.

Imagine a future where a community organizer does not have to spend the first hour of a meeting de-escalating conflict because the participants arrive with the innate ability to regulate their emotions and tolerate ambiguity. Imagine a future where policy makers can debate legislation based on shared facts because their constituents have the critical thinking skills to punish demagoguery and reward nuance. A citizen trained in mentalization does not just vote differently; they relate differently. They enter the workforce, the jury box, and the town square equipped with the psychological resilience to handle difference without collapsing into hatred. By investing in the inner world of the child today, we are, quite literally, building the psychological foundation for every democratic success we hope to achieve tomorrow.

In a world where political discourse is often reduced to a battle of fixed positions, a widespread psychoanalytic education could foster the psychological flexibility needed for democratic deliberation to thrive. It would be a true "ground-up" approach to civic renewal.

Appendix

A Toolkit for the Mentalizing Classroom

This appendix serves as a practical companion to the theoretical frameworks presented in the preceding chapters. While understanding the concepts of mentalization, attachment, and epistemic trust is essential, the translation of these ideas into the daily rhythm of classroom life requires specific strategies and intentional habits. The following toolkit is designed to support educators in bridging the gap between psychoanalytic insight and pedagogical practice. It offers reflective exercises for the teacher, discussion prompts for students, and illustrative case vignettes that contrast non-mentalizing responses with mentalizing interventions. These tools are not intended as a rigid script but rather as a scaffold to support the development of a school culture where the mind is held in mind.

Part I: The Educator's Mirror—Reflective Exercises for Professional Practice

As established in Chapter 8, the educator serves as the primary "mentalizing other" in the classroom. Therefore, the first step in creating a mentalizing classroom is not an external intervention with students but an internal act of calibration by the teacher. These exercises are designed to be used during planning periods, before difficult meetings, or as a decompression ritual at the end of the school day.

Exercise 1: The Preengagement Check-In. Before the school day begins or before a particularly challenging class, take a brief moment to scan your own internal landscape. Ask yourself the following questions: What is my current emotional temperature? Am I carrying residue from a personal interaction or a previous class into this next moment? If I am feeling anxious or irritable, how might that color my interpretation of a student's behavior? This practice engages the self-monitoring function of mentalization. By acknowledging one's own affective state, the educator reduces the likelihood of projecting their own stress onto the students. For example, realizing that one is irritable due to a skipped lunch allows the teacher to pause when a student taps their pencil, recognizing the irritation as internal rather than reacting as if the student is intentionally being provocative.

Exercise 2: Analyzing the Rupture. Conflict and misunderstanding are inevitable in any human environment. When a "rupture" occurs—a moment of conflict, defiance, or disconnection—it is a valuable opportunity for analysis. Instead of focusing solely on the student's behavior, reflect on the mental states involved. Write down or mentally review the incident using these prompts: What did I think the student was feeling in that moment? What did the student think *I* was feeling? Was there a mismatch between my intention and my impact? Did I enter "psychic equivalence," assuming my view of the situation was the only reality? This exercise moves the educator away from a behavioral management mindset, which focuses on compliance, toward a relational mindset, which focuses on repair and understanding.

Part II: Case Vignettes—From Behavior Management to Mentalizing Inquiry

These vignettes illustrate the difference between a traditional, behavior-focused response and a response informed by mentalization theory. The goal in the mentalizing column is not necessarily to "fix" the behavior instantly but to reestablish a connection and understand the internal driver of the action.

Scenario A: The Disengaged Student. *The Situation:* A high school student, usually punctual, has been arriving late and putting their head on the desk for the past week. They refuse to participate in group work.

The Non-Mentalizing Response (Behavioral/Teleological): The teacher assumes the behavior is an act of defiance or laziness. They say, "You need to sit up and pay attention, or I will have to deduct points from your participation grade. It is disrespectful to sleep in my class." *Analysis:* This response focuses entirely on the observable action. It interprets the behavior through a lens of disrespect, likely triggering shame or defensiveness in the student. It fails to wonder about the mind behind the behavior.

The Mentalizing Response (Inquisitive/Attachment-Oriented): The teacher approaches the student quietly during independent work time. They adopt a "not-knowing stance" and say, "I've noticed you've seemed really exhausted this week, which is different from how you usually are. I'm wondering if there is something going on that is making it hard to be here, or if you're just feeling wiped out." *Analysis:* This response validates the observable change without judgment. It offers a tentative hypothesis ("wiped out") but leaves room for the student to correct it. It signals that the teacher is interested in the student's well-being, preserving the attachment bond and inviting the student to share the mental state driving the behavior (e.g., "My parents are fighting," or "I'm working a night shift").

Scenario B: The Polarized Civic Debate. *The Situation:* During a civics lesson on immigration policy, two students begin shouting. Student A claims Student B "hates the country," and Student B claims Student A is "heartless."

The Non-Mentalizing Response (Control-Focused): The teacher intervenes by shouting, "Stop it! We do not yell in this classroom. Both of you are being disruptive. If you can't discuss this civilly, we will move on to the textbook." *Analysis:* This shuts down the affect without processing it. It creates a vacuum where the students' intense emotions remain unresolved, likely reinforcing their belief that the "other side" is impossible to talk to.

The Mentalizing Response (Hot Mentalization/Civic Repair): The teacher pauses the class and lowers their voice to model regulation. "Let's pause. The temperature in the room just went up very high, which tells me you both care deeply about this. Student A, you feel that Student B's view threatens the safety of the country. Student B, you feel Student A's view lacks compassion. Is that right? Let's look at what values are underneath these strong feelings, rather than attacking each other's character." *Analysis:* The teacher names the affect ("temperature went up") and validates the underlying values (safety vs. compassion) without taking a side. By articulating the mental states of both parties, the teacher helps the students see the mind of the other, moving them away from "us vs. them" splitting and toward a more complex understanding of the conflict.

Part III: Classroom Discussion Prompts for Developing Mentalization and Critical Thinking

These prompts can be integrated into existing curricula in English language arts, social studies, and history. They are designed to move students from "what happened" (facts) to "why it happened" (motivations, beliefs, and emotions).

For Literature and Fiction:

- Instead of asking, "What did the character do?" ask: "What belief did the character hold that made them think this action was the only choice?"
- "If we could see this scene from the antagonist's perspective, how might they describe the hero's actions? What would they say the hero is doing wrong?"
- "The character says they are angry, but what other feelings might be hiding underneath that anger? Are they also afraid, embarrassed, or hurt?" (This fosters emotional granularity.)

For History and Civics:

- "When we look at this historical conflict, it is easy to see who was right and who was wrong from our modern perspective. But let's try to imagine the mind of a person living in that time. What were they afraid of? What information did they have, and what information were they missing?"

- "How does this political advertisement try to make you feel? Is it trying to make you feel safe, angry, or proud? Why would the creator of the ad want to trigger that specific emotion in your mind?" (This links mentalization with media literacy.)
- "We often trust information from people who look like us or belong to our group. Can you think of a time you trusted a source just because they were 'on your team'? What does that tell us about how our minds work?"

Part IV: Cultivating the "Not-Knowing" Stance

Perhaps the most powerful tool in the mentalizing classroom is the cultivation of a culture where "I don't know" is viewed as the beginning of inquiry rather than a failure of intellect. In a democratic society, the certainty of one's own righteousness is often the precursor to authoritarianism. To counter this, educators can explicitly model intellectual humility.

- *Model Uncertainty:* When a student asks a complex question, occasionally answer with, "I'm not actually sure about that. I have some thoughts, but I might be missing a piece of the puzzle. What do you all think?"
- *Reward Curiosity over Certainty:* Praise students not just for having the correct answer but for asking a question that reveals a new way of looking at the problem. "That is a fascinating question because it makes us think about what this person was feeling, not just what they did."
- *The "Pause" Button:* Introduce a class signal for when a discussion becomes too heated or confusing. Call it a "mentalizing pause." During this minute of silence, ask students to write down not what they want to say next but what they think the person they disagree with is feeling. This simple mechanical interruption allows the prefrontal cortex to reengage, dampening the amygdala's fight-or-flight response.

By consistently utilizing these tools, educators do more than teach content; they shape the neural and psychological architecture of the next generation. They help build a citizenry that is capable of pausing, reflecting, and seeing the humanity in the other—skills that are the very bedrock of a sustainable democracy.

References

Ainsworth, M. D. S., Blehar, M. C., Waters, E., & Wall, S. (1978). *Patterns of attachment: A psychological study of the strange situation*. Lawrence Erlbaum Associates.

Allen, J. G., & Fonagy, P. (2006). *The handbook of mentalization-based treatment*. John Wiley & Sons.

Anderson, L. W., & Krathwohl, D. R. (Eds.). (2021). *A taxonomy for learning, teaching, and assessing: A revision of Bloom's taxonomy of educational objectives*. Longman.

Bak, P. L., Midgley, N., Zhu, J. L., Wistoft, K., & Obel, C. (2015). The resilience program: Preliminary evaluation of a mentalization-based education program. *Frontiers in Psychology*, *6*, Article 753. https://doi.org/10.3389/fpsyg.2015.00753

Bateman, A. W., & Fonagy, P. (2004). *Psychotherapy for borderline personality disorder: Focusing on mentalization*. Oxford University Press.

Bion, W. R. (1961). *Experiences in groups*. Tavistock Publications.

Bloom, B. S., Englehart, M. D., Furst, E. J., Hill, W. H., & Krathwohl, D. R. (1956). *Taxonomy of educational objectives, handbook I: The cognitive domain*. David McKay Co.

Bowlby, J. (1969). *Attachment and loss, vol. 1: Attachment*. Basic Books.

Bowlby, J. (1988). *A secure base: Parent-child attachment and healthy human development*. Basic Books.

Brackett, M. A., Bailey, C. S., Hoffmann, J. D., & Simmons, D. N. (2019). RULER: A theory-driven, systemic approach to social, emotional, and academic learning. *Educational Psychologist*, *54*(3), 144–161. https://doi.org/10.1080/00461520.2019.1614447

Bretherton, I. (1992). The origins of attachment theory: John Bowlby and Mary Ainsworth. *Developmental Psychology*, *28*(5), 759–775. https://doi.org/10.1037/0012-1649.28.5.759

Cohen, J., McCabe, E. M., Michelli, N. M., & Pickeral, T. (2009). School climate: Research, policy, teacher education and practice. *Teachers College Record*, *111*(1), 180–213.

Durlak, J. A. (2022). *Handbook of social and emotional learning*. Guilford Press.

Durlak, J. A., Weissberg, R. P., Dymnicki, A. B., Taylor, R. D., & Schellinger, K. B. (2011). The impact of enhancing students' social and emotional learning: A meta-analysis of school-based universal interventions. *Child Development*, *82*(1), 405–432.

Facione, P. A., Facione, N. C., & Giancarlo, C. A. (2000). The disposition toward critical thinking: Its character, measurement, and relationship to critical thinking skill. *Informal Logic*, *20*(1), 61–84.

Fonagy, P. (2014). The social context of psychoanalytic therapy: The case of epistemic trust. *Psychology and Psychotherapy: Theory, Research and Practice*, *87*(4), 391–412.

Fonagy, P., & Allison, E. (2014). The role of mentalizing and epistemic trust in the therapeutic relationship. *Psychotherapy*, *51*(3), 372–380. https://doi.org/10.1037/a0036505

Fonagy, P., Gergely, G., Jurist, E. L., & Target, M. (2002). *Affect regulation, mentalization, and the development of the self*. Other Press.

Fonagy, P., Steele, M., Steele, H., & Target, M. (1997). The parent-infant dialogue and the development of the representational world. *Journal of Child Psychology and Psychiatry, 38*(6), 619–631.

Fonagy, P., & Target, M. (1996). Playing with reality: I. Theory of Mind and the normal development of psychic reality. *The International Journal of Psychoanalysis, 77*(2), 217–233.

Gottfredson, D. C., Cross, A., Wilson, D., Rager, O., & Franchino, B. (2010). Effects of the Second Step curriculum on academic achievement and prosocial behavior. *Journal of Research on Educational Effectiveness, 3*(4), 302–332.

Greenberg, M. T., & Jennings, P. A. (n.d.). *CARE: A teacher-focused mindfulness and social-emotional learning program*. Create for Education. Retrieved from https://createforeducation.org/care-an-educator-sel-program-with-proof/

Greenberg, M. T., & Kusche, C. A. (1993). *Promoting Alternative Thinking Strategies (PATHS)*. Developmental Research and Programs.

Grosse, C., Wiesmann, C., & Koch, C. (2017). Training Theory of Mind: A meta-analysis of controlled intervention studies. *Developmental Science, 20*(4), e12465. https://doi.org/10.1111/desc.12465

Humphrey, N., et al. (2018). *The PATHS curriculum for promoting social and emotional well-being among children aged 7–9 years: A cluster RCT*. NIHR Journals Library. Retrieved from https://www.ncbi.nlm.nih.gov/books/NBK519670/

Institute of Education Sciences. (n.d.). *What Works Clearinghouse*. Retrieved from https://ies.ed.gov/ncee/wwc/

Kahan, D. M. (2013). Ideology, motivated reasoning, and cognitive reflection. *Judgment and Decision Making, 8*(4), 407–424.

Lawson, G. M., Bridgeland, J. M., Rofes, E., & Jones, S. M. (2019). *The current state of social and emotional learning implementation in US schools*. American Institutes for Research.

Lecce, S., Cavallini, E., & Pagnin, A. (2014). An innovative European program designed to enhance children's social and emotional learning in preschool settings. *Early Education and Development, 25*(3), 390–405. https://doi.org/10.1080/10409289.2014.821035

Lecce, S., et al. (2017). Enhancing advanced Theory of Mind skills in primary school: A training program. *Child Development, 88*(5), 1546–1559. https://doi.org/10.1111/cdev.12644

Leslie, A. M. (1987). Pretense and representation: The origins of Theory of Mind. *Psychological Review, 94*(4), 412–426. https://doi.org/10.1037/0033-295X.94.4.412

Marttunen, M., Laitila, S., & Lahtinen, T. (2020). Implementing a mentalization-based intervention for early childhood education: The SAGA project. *Early Childhood Education Journal, 48*(4), 481–490. https://doi.org/10.1007/s10643-020-01037-1

Messina, K. E. (2009). Taking back projections: The despair and hope in projective identification. In M. Vardalos (Ed.), *Engaging terror: A critical and interdisciplinary approach*. Universal Publishers, Inc./Brown Walker Press.

Miskowiec, R. A., & Bloom, C. (2016). Improving Theory of Mind in low-income preschoolers: A storybook intervention. *Early Education and Development, 27*(4), 519–532. https://doi.org/10.1080/10409289.2015.1110058

Moy, G. E., & Hazen, A. A. (2018). Systematic review of the Second Step program. *Journal of School Psychology, 71*, 18–41. https://doi.org/10.1016/j.jsp.2018.10.006

Overwalle, F. V. (2008). Social cognition and the brain: A meta-analysis. *Human Brain Mapping, 30*(3), 829–858. https://doi.org/10.1002/hbm.20547

Parsons, S., Gonda, D., & Conway, A. (2017). Virtual reality in social-emotional learning: A pilot study of Theory of Mind training for children aged 5–6. *British Journal of Educational Technology, 48*(2), 374–383. https://doi.org/10.1111/bjet.12466

Paul, R., & Elder, L. (2007). *The miniature guide to critical thinking: Concepts and tools*. Foundation for Critical Thinking Press.

Perron, R. (2014). *The impact of Facing History and Ourselves on students: A summary of research findings*. Facing History and Ourselves. Retrieved from https://www.facinghistory.org/sites/default/files/The%20Impact%20of%20Facing%20History%20and%20Ourselves%20on%20Students.pdf

Proctor, G., Cahill, J., Gore, S., Owen, K., & Rees, A. (2021). A not-knowing, values-based and relational approach to counselling education. *British Journal of Guidance & Counselling, 49*(5), 700–712. https://doi.org/10.1080/03069885.2021.1912289

Schwarzer, N.-H., Dietrich, L., Gingelmaier, S., Nolte, T., Bolz, T., & Fonagy, P. (2023). Mentalizing partially mediates the association between attachment insecurity and global stress in preservice teachers. *Frontiers in Psychology, 14*, Article 1204666. https://doi.org/10.3389/fpsyg.2023.1204666

Schwarzer, N.-H., Heim, N., Gingelmaier, S., Fonagy, P., & Nolte, T. (2024b). Mentalizing as a predictor of well-being and emotion regulation: Longitudinal evidence from a community sample of young adults. *Psychological Reports*. Advance online publication. https://doi.org/10.1177/00332941241261902

Schwarzer, N.-H., Link, P. C., Nolte, T., Turner, A., Kirsch, H., Langnickel, R., & Gingelmaier, S. (2024a). Mentalizing and self-efficacy—disentangling their impact on well-being and symptom severity in novice special education teachers. *European Journal of Special Needs Education*. Advance online publication. https://doi.org/10.1080/08856257.2024.2402167

Spiro, M. E. (1987). *Culture and human nature: Theoretical papers of Melford E. Spiro*. University of Chicago Press.

Stern, D. N. (1985). *The interpersonal world of the infant: A view from psychoanalysis and developmental psychology*. Basic Books.

Streeter, B. (n.d.). *The Alliance for Psychoanalytic Schools: Promotion of psychoanalytic ideas in all schools*. The American Psychoanalyst. Retrieved from https://apsa.org/wp-content/uploads/apsaa-publications/vol54no1-TOC/html/vol54no1_12.xhtml

Thapa, A., Cohen, J., Higgins-D'Alessandro, A., & Guffey, S. (2013). A review of school climate research. *Review of Educational Research, 83*(2), 357–385. https://doi.org/10.3102/0034654313483907

Wellman, H. M. (1990). *The child's Theory of Mind*. MIT Press.

What Works Clearinghouse, WWC. Retrieved from https://ies.ed.gov/ncee/wwc/

Winnicott, D. W. (1971). *Playing and reality*. Tavistock Publications.

Zmigrod, L. (2025). *The ideological brain: The radical science of flexible thinking*. Oxford University Press.

Index

For Product Safety Concerns and Information please contact our EU representative GPSR@taylorandfrancis.com Taylor & Francis Verlag GmbH, Kaufingerstraße 24, 80331 München, Germany